Natural Woman

Look radiant, feel young, beat stress

penelope sach

PENGUIN BOOKS

PENGUIN BOOKS

Published by the Penguin Group
Penguin Group (Australia)
250 Camberwell Road, Camberwell, Victoria 3124, Australia
(a division of Pearson Australia Group Pty Ltd)
Penguin Group (USA) Inc.
375 Hudson Street, New York, New York 10014, USA
Penguin Group (Canada)
90 Eglinton Avenue East, Suite 700, Toronto, Canada ON M4P 2Y3
(a division of Pearson Penguin Canada Inc.)
Penguin Books Ltd
80 Strand, London WC2R 0RL England
Penguin Ireland
25 St Stephen's Green, Dublin 2, Ireland
(a division of Penguin Books Ltd)
Penguin Books India Pvt Ltd
11 Community Centre, Panchsheel Park, New Delhi – 110 017, India
Penguin Group (NZ)
67 Apollo Drive, Rosedale, North Shore 0632, New Zealand
(a division of Pearson New Zealand Ltd)
Penguin Books (South Africa) (Pty) Ltd
24 Sturdee Avenue, Rosebank, Johannesburg 2196, South Africa

Penguin Books Ltd, Registered Offices: 80 Strand, London, WC2R 0RL, England

First published as *Natural Woman* (Penguin Books Australia Ltd 2002)
and *Natural Nourishing Recipes* (Penguin Group (Australia), a division of Pearson Australia Group Pty Ltd 2006)
This revised edition, with additions, published by Penguin Group (Australia) 2008

1 3 5 7 9 10 8 6 4 2

Copyright © Penelope Sach 2008

Design by Megan Baker © Penguin Group (Australia)
All photographs courtesy Digital Vision
Typeset in 11.5/18 pt Tribute by Post Pre-press Group, Brisbane, Queensland
Printed and bound in China by 1010 Printing International Limited

National Library of Australia
Cataloguing-in-Publication data:

Sach, Penelope.
Natural Woman.

New and updated ed.
Includes index.
ISBN 978 0 14 300811 8 (pbk.).

1. Naturopathy. 2. Women – Health and hygiene. 3. Self-care, health. 4. Cookery (natural foods). I. Title.

613.0424

Contents

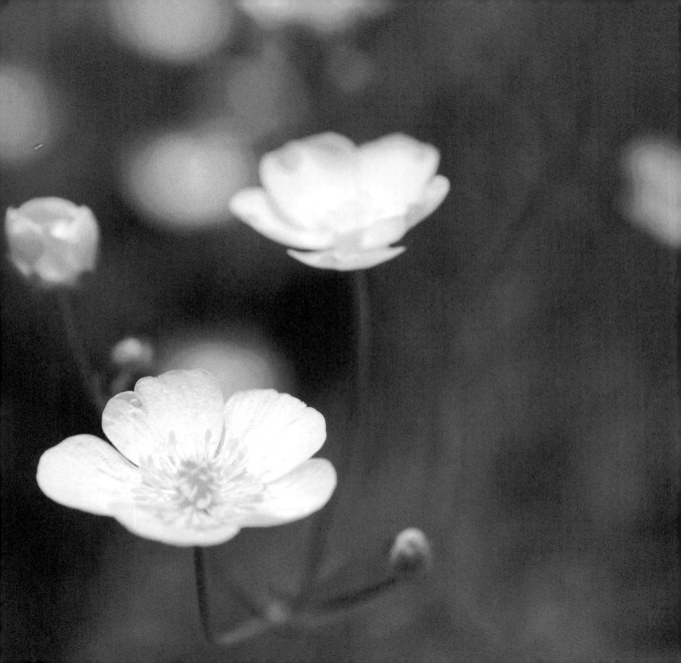

Introduction

Women are truly remarkable. They nurture, they love, they work, they play, they bear children and they are forever balancing their lives with the responsibilities of partners, family, work and friends. Combine these stresses with health and ageing issues, and the modern woman has much to contend with – sustaining good health and ageing gracefully have therefore become a priority.

The women I have treated over the years – many of whom never thought they could achieve great vitality, happiness and balance – are wonderful proof that anything is possible with a little discipline, motivation and organisation.

Self-esteem is essential for women. When a woman's self-esteem suffers, it affects her entire life – not only her health and vitality but also her decision-making abilities, relationships, confidence, career and inner consciousness. Improving self-esteem takes courage, lots of soul-searching and determination. But women are great at this, aren't they? They have a superb ability, once they are motivated, to really change.

As a healer I have observed women regain their self-esteem through improving their physical health. This, in turn, improves their mental health. I often say to my clients, 'Change your eating habits, exercise regularly, and do something spiritually rewarding for yourself and then see what is left over.' Rarely do they have to spend money on long-term counselling. The world opens up to them when they open up to it. Habits are difficult to break but with gradual changes you can reap great rewards.

Natural medicine seems to have a particular significance for women. Traditionally, it was very much part of a woman's domain. Throughout the centuries, women were the gatherers of the seeds, nuts, berries and herbs needed for food and medicines. The knowledge they gleaned has been passed down through the ages in legends, recipes and, of course, 'old wives' tales', many of which have their basis in truth. It's only in the last decade or so that scientists are proving the profound therapeutic effects of many plants and herbs. For example, black cohosh has been found to have powerful properties and can effectively treat menopausal symptoms. It was well known to the American Indians, who used it for this purpose. Similarly, chasteberry (*Vitex agnus-castus*), which was mentioned in the records of Hippocrates in the fourth century BC, is today recognised by the regulating health body of the German government as an effective treatment for abnormal menstrual cycles and premenstrual tension (PMT), and to assist in pre-menopause.

It seems only sensible to turn to these and other natural therapies as an aid to dealing with modern life.

The ten most common questions I am asked are:

- How can I have more energy?
- How can I get to sleep and stop feeling tired?
- How can I lose weight?

- How can I have a flat stomach?

- How can I find time to exercise?

- How can I improve my skin?

- How can I have sparkling eyes?

- How can I strengthen my nails?

- How can I improve my libido?

- How can I improve my memory?

The information in this book will answer these questions, and more. *Natural Woman* is about taking control of your life and making the changes necessary to improve your quality of life.

Adopt the principles in this book and see for yourself that renewed vitality and healthy habits lead to better quality of life. Take up that study you have always wanted to do. Renew old friendships you once cherished. Speak to the man you always admired and tell him so. Take that holiday you always wanted, even if it is for a shorter time than you would like. Change your job if it's really not for you and try something different. Incorporate simple pleasures into your life.

In this new edition I have combined all the information from the original *Natural Woman* with my recipes from *Natural Nourishing Recipes*, and included a new chapter covering the key points of my book *Detox*. I have updated the information where appropriate and worked to ensure this book will help you take control and reap the benefits of a natural approach to healing, health – and life!

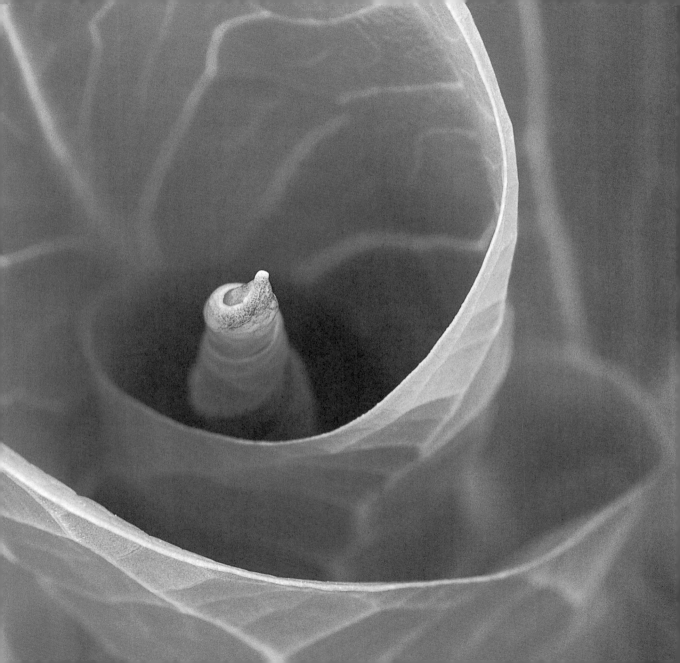

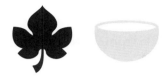

1. Your appearance

Many women I see complain of dull, tired skin, dry hair and brittle, breaking nails. Women prone to these problems are often busy people who don't have a regular, balanced diet. They may be vegetarian and not getting sufficient protein from legumes or they may eat sporadically, skipping lunch or just having a salad with no protein component.

The following are major factors in maintaining healthy skin, hair and nails:

- protein
- calcium
- high fluid intake
- good digestion
- hormonal balance.

Protein

Skin, hair and nails are all made from protein. To regenerate skin tissue, hair follicles and nail beds, a woman's diet must include plenty of protein.

Every day you should eat at least two proteins from the following:

- fish
- chicken
- red meat
- legumes (soya beans, lima beans, adzuki beans, lentils)
- nuts and seeds (especially almonds, sesame seeds and pumpkin seeds)
- eggs (two eggs – or egg whites for people with high cholesterol – every second day)
- cheese
- rice, soya or dairy milk
- yoghurt (a source of light protein).

Note: Drink soya, rice or low-fat milk in between meals or as a protein meal in the mornings. Add yoghurt and blended fruit for a more filling meal.

Calcium

Calcium is essential for skin, hair and nails. If you have eliminated dairy foods from your diet, then a supplement is advisable. Eating a small tub of yoghurt daily is a sure way to obtain calcium. Make sure it contains acidophilus, the friendly bacteria that assists digestion. Low-fat milk or soya milk with added calcium or low-fat white cheese are also good sources of calcium and should be included in your diet daily. However, fermented cheeses such as blue-veined varieties and cheddar can disturb your digestion; avoid them, especially if you are prone to a bloated stomach.

Calcium is also found in almonds and sesame seeds, which make good snacks or can be ground and added to cereal or low-fat milkshakes. The small bones of tinned fish such as salmon and sardines are a good source as well, and so are parsley, watercress, spinach and onions.

High fluid intake

High fluid intake promotes good circulation and hydrates your body, which is vital to the health of your skin, hair and nails. Eight glasses of pure water or herbal tea a day keep nutrients flowing through the blood and clear waste from cell tissues. Water assists the liver and kidneys to remove toxins from the body.

I highly recommend a glass of water with the juice of half a lemon each morning, which acts as a mini-detox for the liver (see Chapter 5, 'Detox', for more about detoxing).

Good digestion

Sit down whenever you eat, and chew slowly. Protein is broken down by saliva and stomach acids, so a rushed meal encourages poor protein digestion and bloating.

Hormonal balance

Fluctuations in hormones during pregnancy, post-natal care, premenstrual tension and menopause often affect a woman's appearance. Dry skin, hair loss and brittle nails can occur at these times, as well as fluid retention, a bloated stomach, tender breasts and sugar cravings.

RECOMMENDATIONS for attaining radiant skin

- Exclude all fried foods, cordials and soft drinks from your diet.
- Cut out all white sugar. Use a little honey or brown sugar instead.
- Eat cold-water fish such as salmon, mackerel or tuna three times a week (essential omega-3 fatty acids return moisture to dry skin).
- Include raw carrot juice daily for the natural vitamin A content, which helps to regenerate skin cells and cleanse the liver.
- Alcohol and caffeine dehydrate the skin. Try to avoid them for at least six weeks and then include only a few cups/glasses twice a week. When you reintroduce coffee into your diet, limit yourself to one a day followed by a large glass of filtered water or herbal tea to cleanse the kidneys.

- During summer try Campari and soda, or gin or vodka and tonic, which are less dehydrating than wine and champagne. Avoid cocktails, because they are loaded with sugar and will upset the acid and alkaline balance of your skin.

If you have extra-dry skin, take two evening primrose oil capsules each morning. You can also take an antioxidant supplement with vitamins A, E and C and extract of green tea once a day.

Teenagers with problem skin

Acne can be a major problem for teenagers during puberty, and adults with a poor diet and/or patterns of acne in their family history. Hormones are the main cause of acne in women. For teenage girls, acne can be an embarrassing and depressing part of growing up. At this age hormones are becoming active and can cause radical changes to moods and skin. Increased oestrogen can clog up the liver pathways, which need natural treatments and natural antibiotic cleansers to keep them clear.

RECOMMENDATIONS for teenagers with problem skin

- Take one chasteberry tablet each morning. This herb will help balance and regulate hormonal cycles.
- Take two garlic oil capsules daily.

- Take two echinacea tablets daily.
- Check iron and vitamin B$_{12}$ levels with your doctor, especially if you're vegetarian.

NUTRITION FOR TEENAGE GIRLS

- Cut out as many fatty foods as possible (to avoid overloading the liver) and include fresh orange and carrot juice daily.
- Cut back on red meats (two to three times a week) and include fish such as salmon and tuna.
- Cut back on soft drinks and drink pure water and fresh juices instead.
- If you like only two or three vegetables, concentrate on eating these daily. (If you are a parent, it is better to work with your teenager than against her, as moods can vary considerably during adolescence.)
- If you are playing lots of sport at school, include one complex vitamin B tablet or food a day for energy and to help clear the liver at a faster rate.

A tonic for skin

Combine equal parts of dandelion, schisandra, artichoke and St Mary's thistle and a flavouring of liquorice or peppermint: take 1 teaspoon two to three times a day.

Eczema

Eczema can be hereditary and is exacerbated by seasonal changes, stress and hormone levels. Generally, the yeast in bread, cheese, wine and vinegar aggravates eczema, as do acidic foods (including orange juice, strawberries and passionfruit), refined sugar and chocolate. A doctor can diagnose specific food allergies, but reducing your intake of these foods should help. Cut out all foods to which you are sensitive or allergic.

If your symptoms worsen at particular times of the year – traditionally during spring or autumn – start your treatment three weeks before the expected onset. Travelling to drier climates or countries can also trigger eczema.

RECOMMENDATIONS for combating eczema

- Take two capsules of omega-3 and -6 fatty acids after each meal, then as your skin improves you may reduce the dosage to three capsules a day.

- To soothe and calm your skin, fill a muslin bag with oats and add it to a warm bath; apply sorbolene cream afterwards.

IF ECZEMA BLEEDS

Take an echinacea tablet three times a day to assist the immune system and a garlic tablet three times a day for its antibacterial properties. If the bleeding is severe, you may need a prescribed antibiotic to get the rash under control, and then use the naturopathic treatment measures.

A tonic to help soothe eczema

Combine equal parts of red clover, dandelion, echinacea, burdock, yellow dock and liquorice. For severe eczema: take 1 teaspoon three times a day.

Sun spots

Spots on the skin are generally a form of sun damage and they are difficult to erase. Skin cancer is common in Australia and can be treated if found through regular checks, so it is important that your doctor checks all spots on your skin regularly for any unusual signs. Minor freckles often become darker when women are taking the contraceptive pill; if this is the case you may wish to find another form of contraception.

FABULOUS FEET

Use a buffer daily under the shower to remove dead skin from the soles of your feet. If you have dry feet, take evening primrose oil or include half an avocado in your diet daily. Take vitamin E (300 IU) daily. If your feet are dry but not itchy, use a rich foot cream such as sorbolene or lanolin, obtainable from your pharmacist.

Psoriasis

This condition is often inherited, and flare-ups can occur when you are stressed, travelling, sleep-deprived or generally run-down, and during seasons when airborne allergens increase histamine levels. You can, however, take preventative measures to decrease the reaction.

Help take the pressure off your immune system by eliminating yeast products – breads, wine and vinegar – and refined sugars and cheese from your diet four weeks *before* spring. In these four weeks take one garlic tablet, two evening primrose oil capsules, two fish oil capsules and one echinacea tablet after each meal. Use a cream rich in vitamin E and aloe vera on your skin. Chamomile cream can also soothe the affected skin.

Hair care

For healthy hair it is important to use a high-quality shampoo and a weekly protein pack on your hair. Try to minimise heavy colourings – discuss alternatives with your hairdresser, such as natural products that don't include bleaches and chemicals. Stress also plays a major part in how your hair looks. Try to eat regular meals and include nourishing snacks such as shakes, protein soups and wholemeal biscuits with some chicken, fish or legumes in your diet.

A high protein intake is essential to remedy brittle and breaking hair follicles. If your hair is dull and dry, you can try a protein drink made from 1 tablespoon of soya, rice or whole milk protein, mixed with water or a milk of your choice. Add 1 teaspoon of acidophilus powder to assist digestion, which facilitates absorption and metabolism of nutrients, and take daily.

RECOMMENDATIONS for healthy hair

- Take 50–100 mg each of calcium, magnesium and zinc daily.
- Take one vitamin B-complex tablet daily.
- The mineral silica is vital for good hair and nails. Chew two small tablets two to three times a day. (Buy the homeopathic forms available from health food stores.)
- Use protein packs on your hair once or twice a week (you can buy these from your pharmacy or hairdresser).

Alopecia

Total or partial hair loss known as alopecia can often happen after the birth of a child or even during pregnancy. Trauma, stress and menopause can also aggravate the condition. I have seen cases of hair loss after car accidents, divorce and the loss of a loved one. Sometimes severe cases are inherited. It is important to boost your immune system at this time (follow the treatment for psoriasis on pages 12–13), and to see a naturopath for individual assessment.

Nail care

Nails are a telltale sign of a woman's health and grooming. If you can, have a regular manicure or set aside time each week to apply a nutrition cream to keep your nails strong and shiny.

RECOMMENDATIONS for healthy nails

- Carry a hand cream in your bag and use it frequently.

- Wear gloves when using cleaning fluids or gardening.

- For very dry nail beds, apply lanolin cream at night. This is good if you have eczema under or around the nail bed.

- Take one acidophilus capsule before each meal to assist the digestion of protein and minerals.

- Take one vitamin B-complex supplement daily if you are stressed or anxious and a nail-biter.

- Take one combination tablet of calcium, magnesium and zinc three times a day until your nails have strengthened.

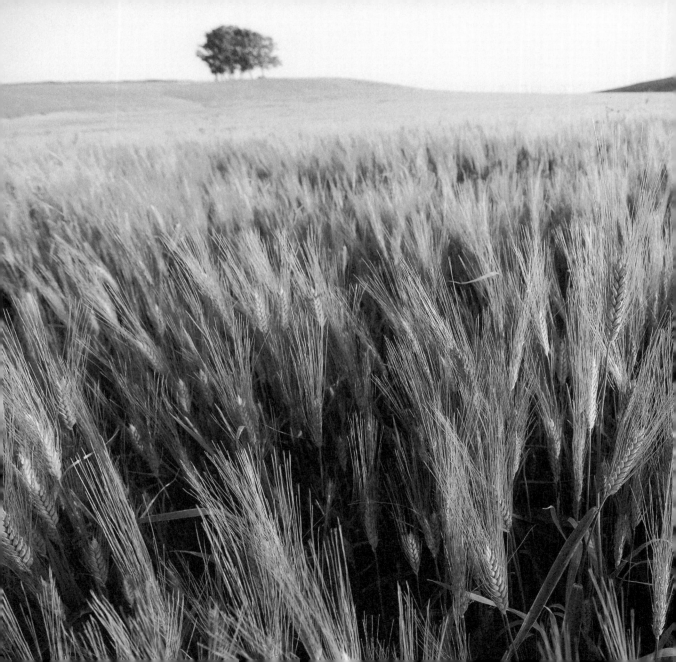

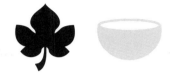

2. Your ideal weight

Women can look fabulous in all shapes and sizes, and most women are happiest when they find their correct weight that allows them to feel and look healthy. Always remember that it is not simply a matter of total weight, but of proportion, and of your inherited bone and body structure. Some women are naturally lighter and slimmer than others. However, all women look radiant and sexy if their bodies are in proportion to their structures.

Whatever you do, don't crash diet. It will only bring long-term disappointment. If you want to lose weight, start by throwing out all the junk food in your cupboards, including cordials, sugary snacks, diet and soft drinks, chocolates, sweet biscuits and white flour products, and hide the alcohol. Have a blood test to check your sugar levels and for diabetes or thyroid problems. If all of these are clear, your lifestyle and habits must be assessed. Poor bowel habits, long-term stress, hormonal imbalance and a history of fad dieting can all be major players when it comes to weight gain.

If you are trying to lose weight or to maintain your ideal weight, there are two critical factors:

- do not undertake quick fixes and/or extreme dieting; and
- be consistent and stick to a healthy eating program, cutting your food intake by 20 per cent.

Weight problems in many women are caused not only by overindulgence in fatty foods but also by an insulin imbalance. Many women eat far too much refined sugar, found in many alcoholic and soft drinks and in foods such as chocolates and biscuits. All these put stress on the pancreas, which has to release insulin to metabolise sugars. A diet high in sugars and carbohydrates causes a critical imbalance, where the body stores sugars as fat rather than burning them up.

RECOMMENDATIONS for assisting weight loss

- Cut right back on white breads, pastries, pasta, biscuits, cakes and refined sugars (for example, in soft drinks and chocolate, and sugar in tea and coffee).
- For healthy bowel flora and regular bowel movements, include 1 teaspoon of psyllium husks on your breakfast cereal. Note that yellow cheeses such as cheddar can cause constipation.
- Include wholemeal fibres on a daily basis: brown rice, grainy wholemeal breads and high-fibre cereal. Also include raw foods such as carrots, lettuce, cucumbers, beetroot and celery in salads or as snacks.

- Eat yoghurt daily that contains acidophilus (a natural flora), which is essential for regulating healthy bacteria in the bowel and therefore in assisting digestion.

- If you crave sugar, try a small snack of Vita-Weat or rye biscuits, or fruit between meals. Yoghurt with fruit will slow down your digestion of the sugar in the fruit.

- Exercise three to four times a week for an hour to keep your metabolism burning unwanted fat.

- Maintain a high fluid intake of filtered water, herbal tea (three to four glasses of each a day) and fresh raw juices (one vegetable or fruit juice daily).

- Eat small meals frequently. Liquid foods such as soup and raw juices also help. Raw or gently steamed vegetables can be eaten any time; they do not add fat or excess fluid.

- Take one to two acidophilus capsules before each meal to assist digestion and ease a bloated stomach.

- Take one B_6 tablet (100 mg) after each meal to assist metabolism and moods and prevent fluid retention.

- Take one chromium tablet (which controls cravings for sugar) after each meal.

- Take one gymnema tablet three times a day to help balance your insulin levels.

Snacks

When you are tempted to reach for sugary snacks, cakes and refined food with hidden fats (butter, chocolate, salami and fried foods), try a snack such as soup, a protein drink, a thin slice of bread or a wholemeal cracker with some low-fat white cheese with honey, or a slice of chicken or ham on a crunchy dry biscuit. (See also the snacks in Chapter 11, 'Natural Nourishing Recipes'.)

SUGAR CRAVINGS

The herb gymnema (*Gymnema sylvestre*) grows in India, Sri Lanka, China, Japan, Malaysia, Indonesia and Vietnam. Its Hindi name means 'sugar destroyer' because it has the amazing property of suppressing cravings for sugar. It is wonderful for those suffering from diabetes and sugar cravings. Ideally, it should be used every two to three hours throughout the day. With a dropper, place 1–2 ml of the liquid extract on the tongue. Leave for one minute then rinse off with water.

A tonic for sugar cravings

Combine equal parts of dandelion root (to clean the liver), bilberry (to normalise blood sugar), St Mary's thistle (to help fat metabolism in the liver) and dandelion leaves (to reduce fluid retention): take 1 teaspoon three times a day in a glass of water for two to three months or until your eating habits have improved and your weight has stabilised.

PROTEIN POWDERS

You may wish to buy a soya protein powder or a rice-based protein powder to use as a quick pick-up drink if you are busy with children or at work. Add 1 heaped teaspoon to a glass of water or low-fat milk. (You can also include a fruit in this drink for flavour and health.)

TEENAGERS WHO DIET

Teenage girls who diet need to take a complex mineral tablet containing calcium, magnesium, zinc and potassium each morning and evening. This is particularly important for adolescent girls between the ages of twelve and eighteen because it is during this time that their bones develop to full strength.

Bloating

Bloating is one of the most distressing and frustrating conditions for women, especially if they do not know how to address it. Generally the two main causes of bloating are an overload of yeast and fermented foods in the diet, and hormonal imbalance, particularly seven to ten days before the period.

RECOMMENDATIONS for avoiding bloating

- Eliminate all yeasty foods (especially bread), pasta, cheese, cakes and biscuits, and refined desserts, chocolate, white sugars, rich sauces and wine from your diet. (You can have two slices of yeast-free bread daily.)

- Make sure you are moving your bowel once a day. If not, include a herbal (senna) laxative with a glass of water at night for six weeks.

- Drink at least eight glasses of pure water daily and include organic herbal teas and one or two raw juices daily (away from food).

- Eat low-fat yoghurt in the morning and at night, or take two acidophilus capsules before each meal, until bloating decreases.

- If you experience premenstrual bloating take two evening primrose oil capsules morning and night.

- Avoid any vitamin or herb that aggravates your digestion.

- Do 20–40 stomach crunches daily to tone stomach muscles (they also tighten the bladder muscles for women). Lie on your back with your knees bent and your feet on the floor. Gently use your stomach muscles to raise your torso towards your knees. Begin slowly and build on these exercises.

Cellulite

This type of fat seems to be connected to hormonal imbalance and inadequate exercise. There is no wonder cream or drug that will fix cellulite. In my experience, the best way of discouraging more cellulite (and reducing what you already have) is to increase your intake of water or herbal tea to at least eight glasses a day. It is also important to exercise three to four times a week. Really do it and don't just think about it – during your 'thinking' time the cellulite is also thinking about getting worse!

Exercise

It is difficult for busy women to include regular exercise in their lives, but it is essential to assist with weight loss and more generally with a sense of wellbeing. You may speed up your diet program by power walking for an hour four times a week. Try to do some form of aerobic exercise two to three times a week. Aerobic classes, swimming, cycling and dancing (anything that increases your heart rate and makes you sweat for an hour) are all good and can be a lot of fun.

Hunger repressants

Do not use hunger repressants – they cause damage to the natural digestive enzymes that are vital in breaking down proteins, fats and sugars. If you have poor digestion, try taking an enzyme tablet (available from health stores) with your meal.

Gluten-free eating

If you are very disciplined, a fast and healthy way to lose weight is to remove gluten from your diet. Gluten is a sticky substance found in most grains except rice and corn, so you must eliminate all breads, pastas, biscuits, croissants, cakes and cous-cous. Sometimes soya products contain gluten. Do this for the time it takes you to achieve your optimum body weight (the weight at which you feel comfortable and healthy). I find that following a gluten-free diet for six to eight weeks has a remarkable effect on weight loss. You may wish to use gluten-free bread or pasta, but you will have better results if you include vegetables, rice and potatoes (for your carbohydrate balance) instead with your choice of protein.

Extreme bloating and bowel irregularities may indicate gluten intolerance. You may either see a doctor to refer you for further tests, or stop eating all gluten products. It can be a difficult program to follow but it's well worth a three-month trial to see how much better you feel and how flat your stomach becomes.

WHEAT GRASS JUICE

This juice is extraordinary. It contains 90 of the 102 possible trace minerals found in rich soil. It is about 20 per cent protein and has trace amounts of B_{12} (excellent for vegetarians and those who lack energy). It contains many digestive enzymes, which are vital to cell function and assist the body to detox from drugs, cancer, hepatitis B, chronic fatigue, metal poisoning, joint problems and all digestive problems. It is best mixed with water or carrot juice because it can make you feel a little nauseous initially due to its powerful antioxidant properties. It is worth it. Persevere. Incorporate 1 teaspoon, fresh or powdered, into your daily diet.

Food intolerance

If you are extremely bloated and suffer constipation and/or diarrhoea and flatulence, you may be allergic to certain foods. Keep a food diary for six weeks by recording each meal you eat and noting any foods that cause you to bloat. Cut these foods out of your diet for the next six weeks and then introduce them one at a time. If you notice that you are aggravated badly after a certain food, you will know to stop it for at least another three months. Try the food again in small amounts, as long as you can tolerate it.

Anorexia and bulimia

These eating disorders occur particularly in young women and are difficult to treat by naturopathic methods alone. The condition is psychological and can be rooted in emotional trauma, peer-group pressure, drug abuse and body image issues. I recommend working with your doctor, psychologist and naturopath.

For anyone who suffers from these conditions, whey powder makes an excellent protein drink that is light and gentle on the stomach. You can also take one multi-vitamin tablet and one calcium tablet (400 mg) daily.

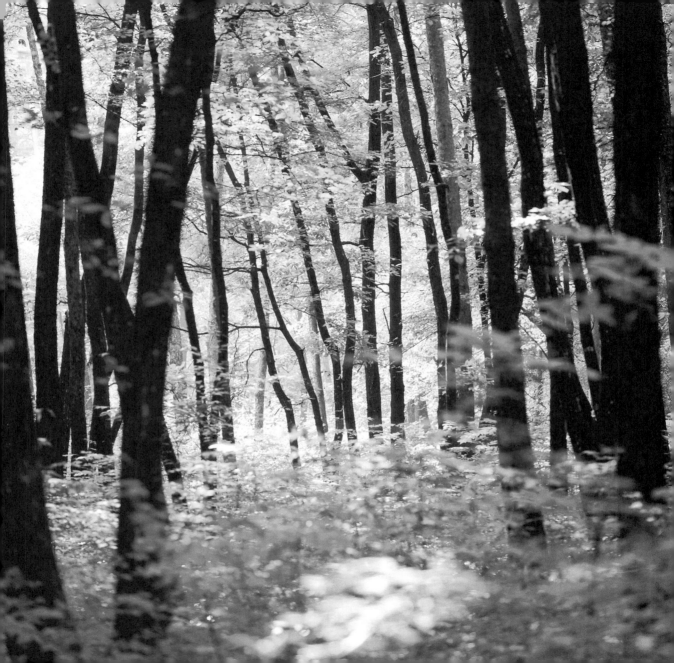

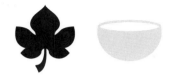

3. Combating stress

Stress, trauma, hormonal imbalance, drug abuse and the pressures of family and work life can all bring about the very real and disturbing symptoms of depression, anxiety and insomnia. These three conditions often go hand in hand, and in the twenty-first century they are a widespread problem that affects women, young and old.

Make a diary of your moods, and see if your mood changes when you eat poorly or around the time of your period. If you're only experiencing these symptoms seven to ten days prior to your period, they could indicate premenstrual tension (PMT).

Sugars leach out important minerals that are essential for the wellbeing of our nerves. One way of keeping depression and anxiety at bay is to avoid the rapid highs and lows following excess sugar intake. Eliminate from your diet all the foods that tend to cause sugar level disturbances, such as sweets, chocolates, cakes, biscuits and alcohol. Also eliminate fried foods, which overload the liver's detoxification pathways. Allergies can often bring on or aggravate mood swings and anxiety attacks, so if you find that certain foods cause these reactions, note this in your diary and eliminate them too. You will be surprised how quickly you can start to take control of your life through these simple measures.

RECOMMENDATIONS for combating stress

- Eat five small meals a day; include in your diet plenty of brown rice, fresh and raw vegetables, fruits, quality proteins such as fish, chicken, eggs, tofu and legumes, and red meat three times a week.
- Eat grainy breads with a protein snack on top to boost your energy.
- Use yoghurt and low-fat milk to boost calcium levels, which settle the nerves.
- Chamomile, petal and vervain tea are traditionally proven to relax and soothe, so drink them throughout the day as well as water and fresh juices.

The feel-good factor

If you are feeling down, talk to your naturopath or doctor to obtain a proper diagnosis. Depression can affect people in different ways and can be hereditary, post-natal, premenstrual, post-traumatic or post-viral, among other causes.

Serotonin is the most important of the feel-good hormones in the brain (Prozac and other antidepressants work on increasing levels of serotonin), and there are ways of increasing this vital hormone naturally, which may help with sadness and depression.

Low melatonin levels are also associated with depression. This natural hormone is produced in deep sleep and has been shown to have healing effects, possibly because when the body is allowed to sleep deeply, the repair of tissues and the immune system can take place correctly. Adequate sleep or melatonin supplements can improve your life dramatically.

A tonic for combating stress

Combine equal parts of St John's wort, Siberian ginseng and panax ginseng, gotu kola and schisandra: take 1 teaspoon two to three times a day for three to six months to help your body increase serotonin and cope with stress. Note: if you are taking antidepressants, you must not take St John's wort.

Exercise

Exercise is vital in the treatment of all forms of depression and anxiety. Research has shown that some form of aerobic exercise for thirty minutes a day (this includes fast walking) increases the production of a vital chemical called phenylethylamine, which is similar in structure to amphetamines (the substances found in antidepressant medication). This natural chemical is sometimes used clinically to treat depression.

In fact, a study at Indiana University concluded that a twenty-minute brisk walk (at a pace that left the person breathing hard but not exhausted) was the best way to boost mental health. The psychological benefits the study discovered were comparable to the sort of improvements expected from a course of psychotherapy.

Anxiety

Many people suffer from anxiety in our hectic world. It can be mild or manifest itself as panic attacks and overwhelming nervousness. It can be a symptom of PMT, experienced seven to ten days before menstruation (see Chapter 6, 'Hormones'). You can take steps to control anxiety, and here are some suggestions for preventing it.

RECOMMENDATIONS for avoiding stress and mood swings

- Diet plays an important role. Eat regular meals, which will keep your blood sugar levels consistent and help prevent mood swings.

- Take calcium and magnesium supplements or eat more yoghurt, low-fat milk and/or cheese, and include almonds and sesame seeds in your daily diet.

- Avoid heavily spiced foods.

- Eliminate caffeine – found in coffee, tea, cola drinks and chocolate – from your diet.

- Do not smoke cigarettes or take recreational drugs.

- During stressful times, watch your breathing. Notice when it becomes quite shallow. Take five to ten deep breaths. This allows more oxygen into your lungs and relaxes your mind.

- A homeopathic remedy called Rescue Remedy is helpful for shock or mild panic attacks during stressful moments. Take five drops every five minutes until you feel better.

- Take one vitamin B-complex tablet once a day.

- Petal, vervain and chamomile tea are wonderful for calming nerves, so drink one of these three times a day.

A tonic for coping with anxiety
Combine equal parts of vervain, passionflower and chamomile: 1 teaspoon in half a glass of water two to three times a day.

Panic attacks

We do not know what causes panic attacks, but we do know they are not all related to stress and anxiety.

Some women have only experienced them after the birth of their children, which could point to hormonal imbalance; other women report experiencing them after a virus, especially if they suffer chronic fatigue. Panic attacks can come at any time, and are often pre-empted by a feeling of overwhelming dread. Your heart rate becomes elevated and you can experience severe sweating.

Treatment for panic attacks varies widely, according to the individual and their circumstances. Worry and anxiety about daily living can be an underlying cause, so if you do suffer from panic attacks, it is important that issues worrying you are addressed. Eliminate as many stressors as possible, and organise your life to help boost your self-esteem and bring you happiness. This could include allowing yourself more time to socialise, indulge in a hobby or exercise.

Natural remedies also have a place in the treatment of panic attacks and it is often wise to try them before resorting to stronger medication.

RECOMMENDATIONS for dealing with panic attacks

- Magnesium, a muscle relaxant, is vital in the treatment of panic attacks, regardless of their cause: take a tablet of 100 mg chelated magnesium, three times a day.

- Take one to two St John's wort tablets a day. (Check with your doctor if you are on other medication.)

- Put five drops of Rescue Remedy (a homeopathic medicine made from the essence of flowers) under the tongue every five minutes during a panic attack.

- Calcium is essential for nerves and should be supplemented, especially if you are not eating many calcium-rich foods. Begin with 500 mg a day and increase the dosage according to advice from your doctor or naturopath.

- Evening primrose oil is useful in some cases, especially if panic attacks occur a week before the start of your period: 3000 mg a day.

- Slow breathing exercises during a panic attack can be miraculous. Take ten deep breaths to slow down your heart rate.

- Regular yoga classes can assist.

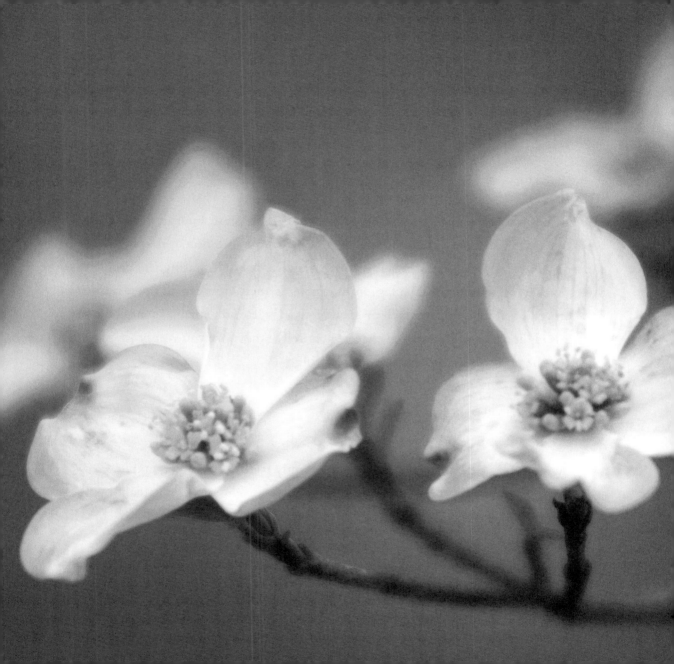

- Pursue new hobbies, contact old friends and instigate a change of job or even a change of environment such as moving house. A great holiday can help relieve accumulated stress.

Insomnia

Sleeping patterns depend very much on your psychological state, but there are natural ways to ensure you have a good night's sleep. It's simply a question of making subtle shifts in your daily routine and being aware of what may be causing the problem. Stress, worry, anxiety, exams, jet lag, sinus problems and illness can all cause insomnia. Going to bed on a full stomach or soon after a large meal can also contribute to a restless night. Insomnia can often exacerbate itself – the more you worry about not sleeping, the more you'll be kept awake worrying.

RECOMMENDATIONS for a sound sleep

- Avoid caffeine – coffee, tea, chocolate – six hours before bed.

- Avoid eating a heavy meal before bed. Eat only freshly cooked vegetables with fish or a light white meat protein. Red meat, rich sauces and alcohol will stimulate digestion and the mind. If you eat these foods, have them three to four hours before bed.

- Try a calcium tablet (500 mg) before bed. Often this will change your sleeping habits by relaxing your nerves.

- Have a cup of organic chamomile tea half an hour before bed to relax your body.

- For persistent insomnia, try one to two Mexican valerian tablets with a glass of warm skim milk or chamomile tea twenty minutes before bed.

- Melatonin assists many people; take one (3 mg) tablet before bed. (In Australia you can only buy melatonin in a homeopathic form, which is not as effective as the 3 mg tablet form. You can, however, ask your doctor to prescribe the tablet for you.)

- In the hour before bed, avoid the mental stimulation of working on a computer or watching television. Twenty minutes of quiet time and meditation during that hour can be very helpful if you suffer from stress.

A tonic to help you sleep

Combine equal parts of chamomile, kava kava, vervain, passionflower: take 1 teaspoon in warm milk or water half an hour before bed.

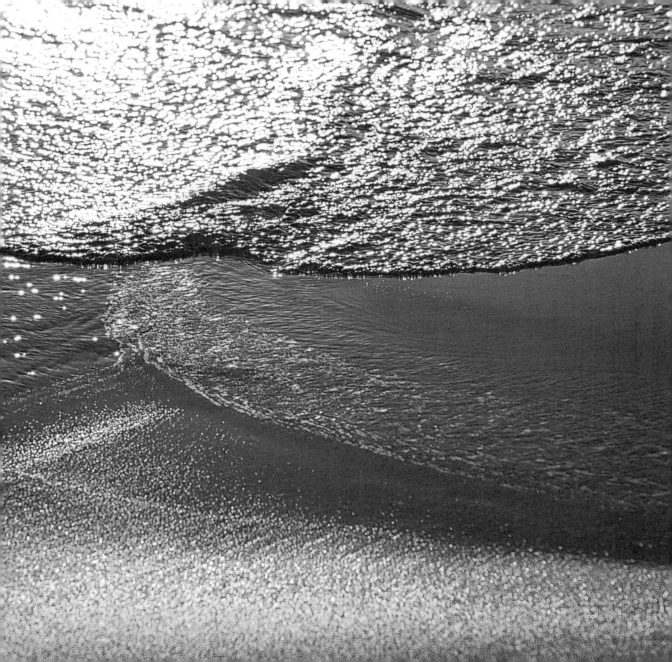

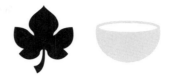

4. Boosting your immune system

Whether you suffer mildly or severely from a depleted immune system, it is essential that you boost your immunity before the onslaught of winter or travel to a colder climate. If you have suffered from major bronchial and asthmatic problems it may take two winters for your system to strengthen, but rest assured that preventative measures do work. With a few simple daily routines, your quality of life can be so much greater.

Signs that your natural immunity is low are regular colds and flus, bronchitis, allergies, asthma, sinus problems, dermatitis (skin irritations) and cystitis.

RECOMMENDATIONS for boosting your immune system (begin the following program four weeks before winter sets in).

- Drink a glass of warm water with freshly squeezed lemon juice (and honey if desired) every morning.
- Drink a freshly squeezed orange juice daily to build vitamin C levels.

- Stay away from mucus-forming foods, such as milk and cheese, and large quantities of bread (use brown rice instead), soft drinks, chocolate and cakes.
- Eat as many fresh vegetables and fruits as you can daily, and include fish high in omega oils (salmon, tuna or sardines) three times a week. They are good for preventing chest complaints.
- Eat thick homemade soups with fresh vegetables, barley and split peas.
- Use garlic and onions as frequently as possible, and include horseradish when you can.
- Include spices, especially ginger and cayenne, in your food.
- Drink peppermint, fresh mint or ginger tea daily.
- Keep alcohol to a minimum, especially champagne and white wine, which are high in additives and can trigger asthma attacks.
- Make sure your iron levels are not low. Ask your doctor for a check well before winter.
- One combination garlic and horseradish tablet after each meal will assist sinus sufferers.
- Take one vitamin C tablet with bioflavonoids (500 mg of each) twice a day.
- Take an immune-boosting tablet made from either echinacea, cat's claw, astragalus and andrographis or any combination. Ask your health store for this supplement. These herbs work in combination to maintain a healthy immune system and fight viral and bacterial infections. Take one tablet, twice a day.

ASTRAGALUS (*ASTRAGALUS MEMBRANACEUS*)

This is an official herb in Chinese and Japanese pharmacopoeias, and it grows well in the mountainous districts of Iran and Iraq. In Chinese medicine astragalus is well respected as a tonic to assist qi (energy) and blood (nutrition). In the western world it is used for treating long-term chronic infections. It boosts the immune system after chemotherapy, radiotherapy and surgery.

RECOMMENDATIONS for fighting a cold

- Make a drink of hot water, lemon juice, honey and freshly grated ginger (1 teaspoon) and drink at least four to five times a day while you are in the severe stages of the flu, and then two to three times a day for a week later.

- Keep fluids high (see previous point) and include hot peppermint tea.

- Use inhalations of peppermint and eucalyptus oils or simply rub some old-fashioned Vicks VapoRub into the chest area regularly.

- Stay in bed and rest for at least twenty-four to forty-eight hours. You may sweat, which is a good sign.

- Take two echinacea tablets after each meal for four days and then four tablets a day until your symptoms improve.

- Take one vitamin C tablet with bioflavonoids (500 mg of each) every three to four hours.

An amazing flu tea

This tea is excellent for fighting colds, flus and fevers. It's safe for everyone over the age of five. Combine the following dried herbs, obtainable from health stores:

- 2 tablespoons yarrow
- 2 tablespoons peppermint
- 2 tablespoons eyebright
- 1 teaspoon ginger
- 1 teaspoon cinnamon
- ½–1 teaspoon cayenne powder

Add 1 teaspoon of the mixture to a cup of boiling water. Drink hot with honey as often as possible.

Virus

Generally symptoms of a virus in the upper respiratory area include a red raw throat, headaches, lethargy and aching muscles. If you have any of these symptoms you should consult your doctor, but for a simple flu virus – if you have a sore throat and lethargy but no runny nose – the following can assist.

RECOMMENDATIONS for fighting a virus

- Rest in bed.
- Drink plenty of fluids, especially fresh fruit juice, water and green tea.
- Eat light food such as soup and cooked vegetables.

- Take vitamin C: 1000 mg every two to three hours.

- Take the herb astragalus – two tablets twice a day until you feel better.

CAT'S CLAW (*UNCARIA TOMENTOSA*)

This is one of the most celebrated plants of the Ashaninka Indians, the indigenous people of the Peruvian central rainforest. Cat's claw became a threatened species in 1994 due to its popularity as an immune-enhancing herb, especially for HIV infections, carcinoma and auto-immune disorders; it is now protected by special legislation in Peru. It is illegal to harvest or disturb the root, so we use the stem bark. Cat's claw is wonderful for post-viral conditions such as chronic fatigue and long-term flu and viral infections. I find it works very well with echinacea and astragalus.

Mouth ulcers and cold sores

Mouth ulcers and cold sores are classic signs that you are generally run-down. They can also indicate that your system is too acidic.

RECOMMENDATIONS for treating mouth ulcers and cold sores

- Eliminate from your diet citrus fruits, tomatoes, wine, white sugar, spices and soft drinks.

- Build your immune system by taking one echinacea tablet each day for three to four months.

- Take a multivitamin with added minerals and an antioxidant tablet.

- For ulcers, combine 2 ml each of myrrh and sage with warm water, then gargle and spit it out. Repeat three times a day.

- For cold sores, dab some liquid extract of *Melissa officinalis* on the affected area three to four times a day. It works quickly to dry it up.

Sinus conditions and hayfever

Seasonal changes can have a profound effect on how you feel. Pollens are a real problem and they quickly cause a histaminic reaction. Pollens irritate the lining of the nose and sinuses; the body compensates by producing phlegm or mucus. Symptoms include sneezing, sinus problems, earaches, coughs and bronchial conditions, dizziness, skin rashes, flaky scalp, dry fingernail beds, red and puffy eyes and general lethargy.

RECOMMENDATIONS for fighting sinus conditions and hayfever
Three weeks before the seasonal changes, take the following steps to build up your immune system.

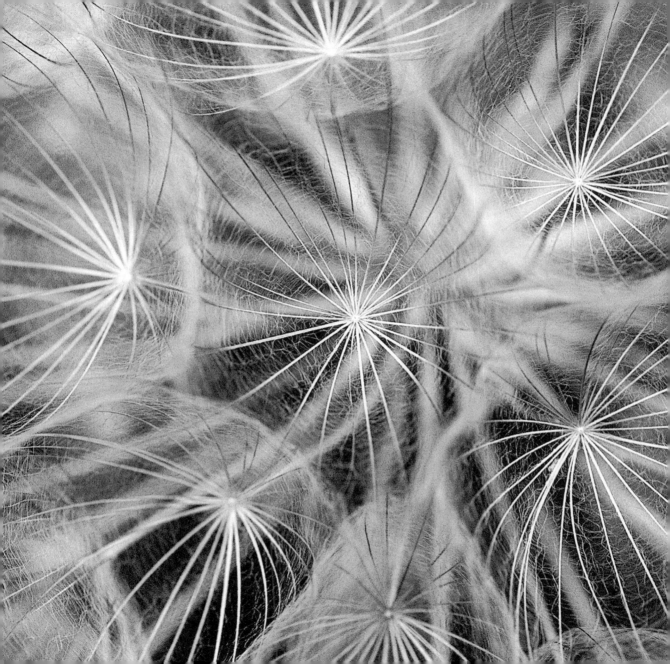

- Wine can aggravate symptoms, so keep your intake to a minimum during high-allergen seasons.
- Take vitamin C with bioflavonoids (500 mg of each): one combination tablet or 1 teaspoon of powder in a glass of water or juice two to three times a day. This strengthens the mucous membranes against airborne foreign bodies in the sinus.
- Take one echinacea tablet after each meal to boost immunity.
- Take one garlic, horseradish and fenugreek tablet after each meal. The garlic acts as a natural antibacterial agent, helping to keep the sinus passage and ears clear of infection.
- Drink lots of fresh orange, pineapple and lemon juice daily: 500 ml of fresh citrus juice a day is ideal during spring.
- Drink three cups a day of ginger and peppermint teas, either combined or by themselves. You may add chamomile, which is excellent for allergies, too, and especially relaxing in the evening.

Airborne allergens

Keep dust from building up around the house, especially in sleeping areas. There are special house 'dust busters' that you may wish to invest in if your family suffers from allergies and asthma. Use environmentally friendly household cleaning agents, particularly those containing eucalyptus oil.

RECOMMENDATIONS for fighting airborne allergens

- Take vitamin C with bioflavonoids (500 mg of each): two tablets or 1 teaspoon of the powder in water every three to four hours during the day for the first forty-eight hours. When you feel better, use this dose two to three times a day.

- Take one euphrasia tablet after each meal. This herb is excellent for hay fever and sinus problems.

- Take two garlic and horseradish tablets (with fenugreek if you can obtain this at your health store) after each meal until you feel better, then lower the dose to one tablet after each meal.

- If you have skin rashes, include two to three evening primrose oil capsules after each meal.

- Place a few drops of peppermint or eucalyptus oil on a cotton handkerchief and breathe it regularly to keep the nasal passageways clear from airborne pollens.

- Ask your local chemist for some soothing eye drops for dry and itchy eyes: use three to four times a day.

- You can use a salt spray in your nose.

A tonic for nasal congestion

Combine equal parts of echinacea, peppermint, elecampane, eyebright, thyme, wild cherry and marshmallow: take 1 teaspoon in water three to four times a day.

Asthma

Asthma can be triggered by many different things. Some sufferers are allergy-prone, others are subject to a general weakness of the immune system – and some are both. A naturopath and herbalist can often get to the source of the problem and can suggest natural vitamins and herbs that can be taken alongside any prescription medicine from your doctor. Remember it is always wise to let your doctor know what supplements you are taking.

RECOMMENDATIONS for combating asthma

- Eliminate any allergy-causing foods from your diet – you may need to consult your doctor or naturopath.
- Dust mites can trigger allergies, so try to minimise dust in your home. Wooden floors are preferable to carpets, and also check whether you have any privet trees in your yard (the pollen can be a problem).
- Use organic chemical-free washing powders, detergents and soaps.
- Keep your stress levels to a minimum by getting plenty of sleep and exercising regularly – swimming can improve lung capacity, so try to swim in salt water (or pools with low levels of chlorine) two to three times a week.
- Throughout winter, take two echinacea tablets a day.
- Take vitamin C with bioflavonoids: 1 teaspoon of powder in juice twice a day.

A tonic for soothing asthma

Combine equal parts of liquorice, thyme, andrographis, echinacea and boswellia: take 1 teaspoon twice a day throughout winter or when your asthma is aggravated.

ANDROGRAPHIS (*ANDROGRAPHIS PANICULATA*)

Traditionally known as the 'king of bitters' in India where it is highly valued as a medicine, this herb is classed as a cold remedy and therefore used to clear heat from the body, especially in the lungs and respiratory organs. It has excellent anti-inflammatory properties and works well in counteracting bacterial and viral infections such as the common cold and viral throats and fevers. Andrographis has been found to be very helpful when used long term against stubborn urinary tract infections. Do not use during pregnancy.

Food intolerances and allergies

After eating certain foods, you may experience an upset or bloated stomach, diarrhoea, skin rashes or itchiness, tiredness, irritability, anxiety, moodiness, constipation or shortness of breath. If symptoms are constantly severe after the same foods, you may have a food allergy. If they are mild and don't happen all the time, it could be a food intolerance. A blood test from your doctor or specialised allergy clinic will help diagnose any allergies. To recover from a food allergy you have little choice but to stay away from the food in question. With a food intolerance, you should be able to eat small amounts of the offending food every three to four days without suffering a reaction.

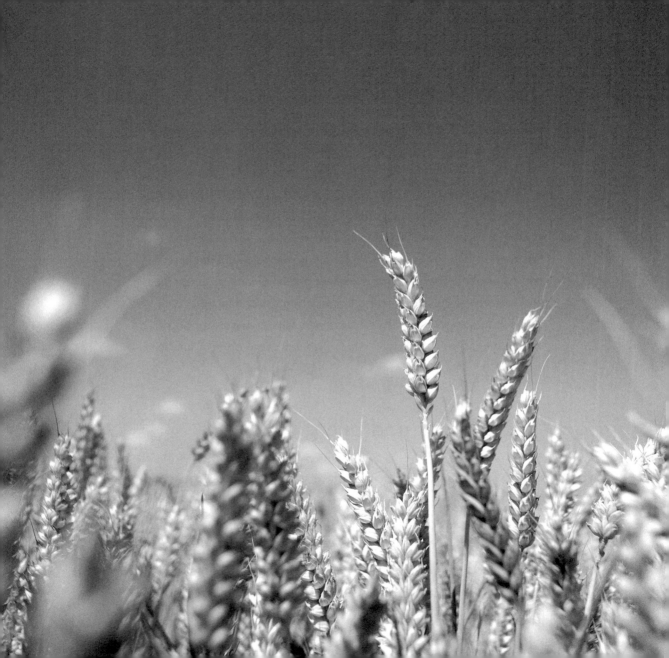

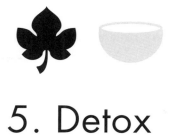

5. Detox

The most common complaint I hear from women is about overwhelming tiredness, chronic fatigue or a general feeling of being run-down. I always recommend a detox program, because it is the essential first step in establishing a pattern of wellbeing and vitality, and can be the start of a new life.

Detoxification means different things to different people. Generally, we understand the word to indicate that there are toxins or poisonous substances in our systems – which can cause physical, and often psychological, distress – that need to be eliminated. The process of detoxification, which has been practised in varying forms for centuries, is often referred to as cleansing the body or purifying the bloodstream.

There is a widespread perception that the body accumulates poisons simply from the rigours of everyday living, and that we need to cleanse these toxins from the body regularly to maintain optimum wellbeing. One of the problems for modern women is that our lifestyles are so hectic – there is barely enough time to think about detoxing, let alone clearing the time to put a detox program into action.

Many of us imagine wistfully that we could do some form of purification in our holiday period, but this is also a time when we like to rest and indulge a little in the foods that we so enjoy. With this in mind, I have created a three-day detox program that is simple and achievable, and allows you to carry out a physical 'clean-up' and gain a resurgence of energy (see page 54).

If you are on any medication, do not undertake any detox program without first consulting your doctor.

What is a toxin?

A toxin is a substance to which the body reacts adversely. Toxins can cause minor problems such as a skin rash, or major ones such as cancer. They are everywhere in our daily lives, from the pollution in the air we breathe to the chemicals that are formed in our bodies from the breakdown of food.

Then there are toxins from the substances that we purposely put in our bodies, such as cigarette smoke, recreational drugs, alcohol, sugar, animal fats and processed food. Thousands of toxins are formed in the bacterial breeding ground of our large intestine, where they multiply at a rapid rate if your diet is poor.

Toxins can develop on our food before we even consume it; bacteria will breed on food that has been kept too long in the refrigerator; and food can ferment in heat and unsuitable packaging. On the other hand, preservatives used to prevent food deteriorating can also be harmful to us when present in large doses.

Acid and alkaline foods

The main causes of acid build-up in the digestive system are:

- poor digestion
- eating proteins and starches together frequently
- eating too much meat
- eating too many refined carbohydrates, including white flour and refined sugar products
- a lack of fresh fruit and vegetables in your diet.

In today's fast-paced world of eating on the run and quick, easy meals, our diets tend to be more acidic than alkaline. When our bodies become too acidic, our system to uses up all the reserves of minerals such as calcium, magnesium, potassium, sodium and iron. These minerals are essential for a healthy nervous system and for strong bones, joints and muscles.

Acid builders

- Refined sugar and white flour products
- Meat
- Alcohol
- Stress

Alkaline builders

- Fresh fruit and vegetables
- All raw juices, especially carrot, watermelon and green vegetable juices (spinach, beetroot greens and wheat grass)
- Herbal teas
- Unpasteurised honey
- Raw almonds
- Miso soup
- Tofu
- Sea vegetables
- Lima and adzuki beans (other beans, except for those that are soaked and have sprouted, are acidic)

Natural detox systems

The body has its own ways of detoxing naturally. The liver acts as a purifying filter for the blood. The gall bladder assists the liver and also breaks down fats. The kidneys eliminate unwanted elements (such as excessive uric acid, proteins and bacteria) in our body. The bowel eliminates unwanted waste, bacteria and toxins from the break-down of our foods. Without these systems working properly together, we would be walking toxic bombs. We would suffer toxaemia (blood poisoning) very quickly and become prey to other life-threatening diseases.

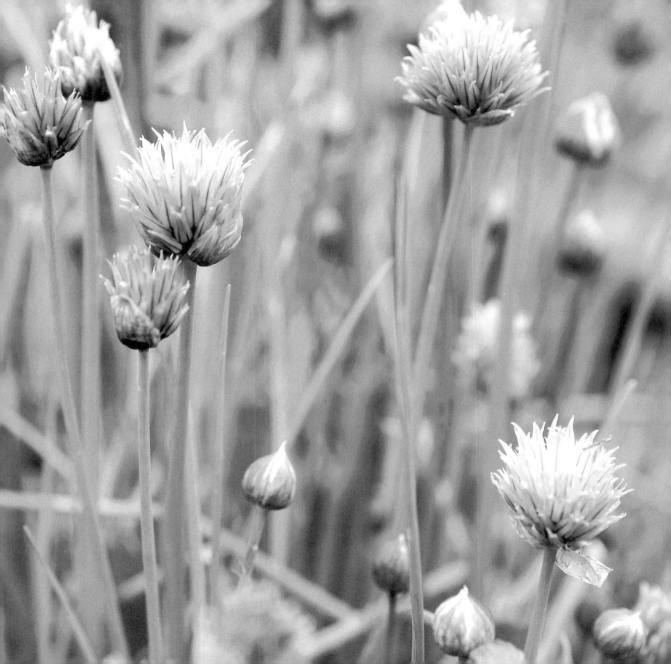

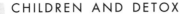

CHILDREN AND DETOX

Children under twelve should not detox. It is very difficult for
a child to change habits overnight, so begin by modifying their
diet to slowly introduce alternative foods without colourings
and preservatives.

A three-day detox

You can undertake a three-day detox once a month to rest your body, or while you
are on holiday or taking some time off work. This three-day detox is safe and simple,
and encourages you to focus on fresh, unrefined foods. In terms of how you will feel
during the detox, the worst period is usually in the first forty-eight hours; after this
you can expect to feel renewed vigour. Less frequently, muscle and joint pain can
occur, and occasionally, skin breakouts. In a three-day cleanse these issues are usually minor, so remember that they will pass, and look forward to the renewed energy
after the hard work.

During the three days, follow these guidelines for your detox.

- Make a soup of parsley, onions, carrots, turnips, zucchini, broccoli and
  cauliflower. Eat a large bowl or cup (at least 300 ml) of this soup every
  two hours of your waking day for the three days.

- If you crave fruit, eat a whole piece – the only fruits allowed are an orange,
  apple or pear – every alternate hour from the soup. (This three-day detox
  does not allow fruit all day because fruit can cause an imbalance in the sugar

levels of the body, leading to highs and lows. Although vegetables also contain natural sugars, they do not overload the body and cause these highs and lows.)

- On each of the three days drink only two glasses of raw carrot juice mixed with beetroot or a green vegetable such as spinach or lettuce.

- On each of the three days drink 2 litres of pure spring or filtered water – one glass every hour. (A glass of water every hour will cleanse your body from the overload of sugar in your system.)

- Rest for at least two hours a day on each of the three days. Do not undertake any exercise more strenuous than light walking. Never use a sauna or steam room during the detox; fainting or nausea can result. The body does not cope well with too many extremes at once.

- You may feel some form of headache, fatigue, weakness in the limbs or mental vagueness. If you develop a strong headache, you can replace the soup with (or eat alongside the soup) raw vegetables such as celery and carrot sticks or some lightly steamed vegetables such as carrots, broccoli, zucchini, spinach and sweet potato, for a more alkaline effect from the detox.

- Don't smoke, drink alcohol or take recreational drugs during the detox.

- Don't take vitamin supplements during the detox. If you are constipated, take 1 teaspoon of vitamin C powder in a glass of water three times a day; or 1 teaspoon of psyllium husks twice a day; or 1 teaspoon of vegetable oil two to three times a day.

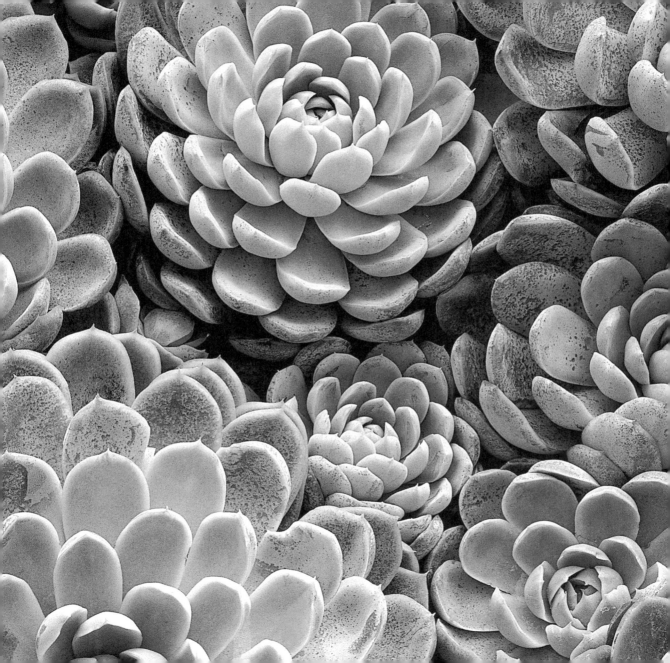

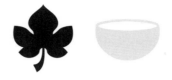

6. Hormones

Very few women are fortunate enough to go through life without some sort of hormonal imbalance. Some women don't realise that their moods and irritabilities are closely related to their monthly cycle. In order to regulate hormones, you must be aware of how your body feels. Beginning on the first day of your period, keep a daily diary of moods, weight fluctuations, breast soreness and anxiety in relation to your cycle. Your cycle could be between twenty-eight and thirty-two days; some women's cycles follow no particular pattern. Through the diary you can monitor how you are affected physically and mentally at different times.

Knowing your cycle

Generally a woman ovulates between the tenth and seventeenth day of her cycle; it is around this time she is most fertile. To work out when ovulation occurs, deduct fourteen days from the first day of your last period. For example, if your cycle is thirty days and your periods are always regular, you will ovulate around day sixteen.

RECOMMENDATIONS for balancing your hormones

- Sugar cravings often happen before a period. For ten days before your period, eat small snacks every few hours or have five to six a day.

- Avoid or eliminate cakes and biscuits containing refined sugar. Eat a piece of fruit instead or a protein snack such as a nut spread on a Ryvita biscuit, a muesli bar or a handful of almonds with a tub of yoghurt.

- Make simple carbohydrate snacks for those times when you crave heavy starches. Keep some thick barley and vegetable soups in the freezer for quick reheating. Cook a potato and add a filling of avocado or tuna with tomato, basil and onions.

- Yeasty foods such as breads, pasta and cakes will aggravate a puffy stomach.

- Make sure you eat fresh vegetables daily in a range of colours. Raw vegetables are also a great snack; dipped in a hummus paste, they can soothe the cravings of the monthly cycles.

- Drink carrot juice with added ginger (ginger helps relieve period pain). Drink fresh juices, water and herbal teas instead of cordials and soft drinks.

- Eliminate cigarettes and caffeine and reduce alcohol to a minimum (three to four glasses per week).

- Wine and champagne contain high levels of sugars and yeast. We often crave these drinks before a period, but try substituting them with vodka and tonic or Campari and soda, which contain little or no sugar and yeast. Fruit cocktails with an alcohol base are deadly before a period.

PMT

Premenstrual tension (PMT) is the name for a condition with a variety of symptoms, including irritability, depression, headaches, fluid retention and breast tenderness, occurring seven days to two weeks before a period. Some women find their lives are severely affected by these difficult symptoms. The liver plays an important role in clearing excess oestrogens in the blood, so decreasing the load on your liver by reducing caffeine and alcohol intake, and taking a vitamin B-complex supplement will assist in the removal of excess oestrogens.

RECOMMENDATIONS for dealing with PMT

- Take 50 drops of chasteberry each morning in half a glass of water, beginning fourteen days prior to your period. Take one tablet each day if you prefer.

- Essential fatty acids in the form of evening primrose oil and fish oil are helpful. Take one capsule of each three times a day, beginning fourteen days prior to your period.

- Magnesium helps relax the muscle tissue of the uterus and ease discomfort. Take 1 teaspoon of magnesium twice a day or one tablet (200 mg) three times a day, beginning fourteen days prior to your period. If you have pain or very severe irritability, take one tablet (200 mg) every four hours.

- If you eat very few foods containing calcium and suffer from insomnia before a period, take 500–1000 mg of calcium before bed. This not only soothes the nerves but is a wonderful sleeping aid.

- During the premenstrual phase depression can be a significant issue because serotonin levels can drop. Take two St John's wort tablets a day to combat symptoms of depression, combined with exercise and rest. Do not take St John's wort if you are taking antidepressants.

- If you have tender or swollen breasts, take vitamin B$_6$ (300–600 mg daily), which can reduce the swelling before a period.

CHASTEBERRY (*VITEX AGNUS-CASTUS*)

Research has shown that this herb enhances corpus luteal development, correcting a progesterone deficiency indicated with PMT. It also normalises the menstrual cycle and encourages ovulation. Note: chasteberry should not be used if you are taking the contraceptive pill.

Period pain

Period pain usually begins on the first day of the period and stops twenty-four hours later. Young women often experience this problem, and it frequently ceases after the birth of a child. In many cases, the pain responds very well to natural medicine. If you have little or no results from this treatment, you can discuss with your doctor the options of pain killers or the contraceptive pill, which can relieve severe symptoms.

RECOMMENDATIONS for dealing with period pain

- Take one magnesium tablet (200 mg) every one to two hours for severe pain.

- Drink ginger tea every hour.

A tonic for easing period pain

Combine equal parts of cramp bark, blue cohosh, black cohosh, dong quai and peppermint: take 1 teaspoon four times a day or every four hours. Ginger should be added if you are not drinking ginger tea. Add 10 per cent ginger to the tonic because this herb is very strong and spicy when taken in concentrated amounts. This tonic can be taken three times a day for a week before your period commences, as it often eases the severity of the pain. It is excellent for teenagers who are too young to take the contraceptive pill.

Heavy bleeding

Often heavy bleeding is a symptom of hormonal imbalance; therefore, maintaining a healthy lifestyle is an essential part of managing this discomfort. You should be examined by a gynaecologist to make sure you have no fibroids or other problems with your uterus.

Note: Some women miss several periods during times of high stress, travel, heavy exercise or extreme dieting. If you are not having periods and are sure you are not pregnant, try the following.

- Have your iron and B_{12} levels checked.
- Take one vitamin B-complex tablet daily.
- Take evening primrose oil: 3000 mg daily.
- Ensure you have a regular protein intake.

Adolescent hormones

It is quite common for a young girl beginning to menstruate to have irregular cycles. A healthy diet is important, but unfortunately it can be hard to influence teenagers' eating habits. However, if your teenager will follow even 70–80 per cent of a healthy diet, supplements can be cut to a minimum. Supplements are tremendous for that extra boost of vitality and for performing well at school.

RECOMMENDATIONS for a girl's first period

- Take two evening primrose oil capsules each morning, which assist the balance of hormones and skin.
- Take one vitamin B-complex tablet after breakfast.
- Take a complex mineral supplement containing calcium, magnesium, zinc and trace minerals: one tablet in the morning and one in the evening before bed. This last dose assists sleep and helps strengthen bones. Calcium is laid down in the bones in adolescents between the ages of twelve and eighteen, and it is essential that calcium supplements (500 mg) are taken daily.

- Iron and folic acid are vital for energy and regular cycles. For young girls who are vegetarian, an iron tablet can be beneficial. If preferred, a tonic of iron-rich herbs is also obtainable at health stores: take 1 teaspoon once to twice a day.

- Skin breakouts often occur at the onset of menstruation. Take one echinacea tablet each morning, beginning a week before each period, to assist in keeping the blood cleaner and boost immunity, which is often lowered at this time.

- Even though fish oils are helpful in regulating PMT, sometimes they can aggravate breakouts in the skin. I recommend increasing fish in the teenager's diet with tins of salmon and fresh fish three times a week.

- Carrot juice is full of antioxidants and excellent for the skin. A glass daily is ideal.

Note: If your teenager plays sport regularly, take them for a blood test to check their iron levels every six months.

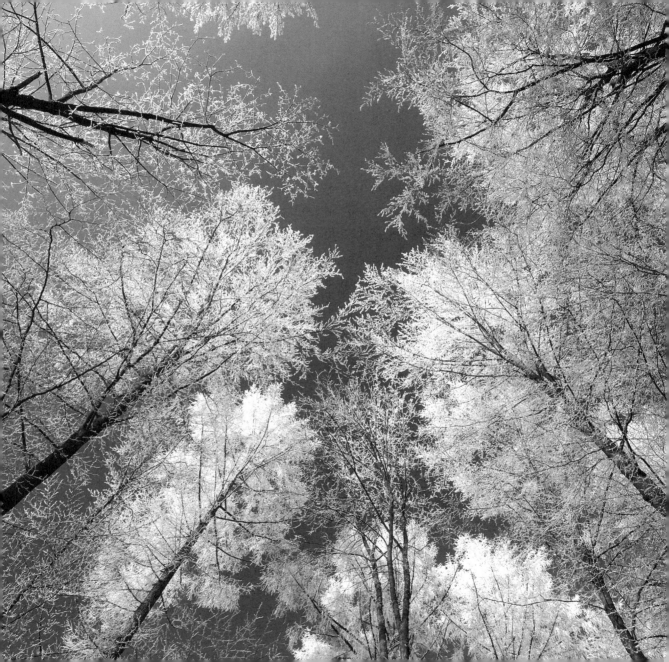

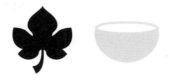

7. Menopause

Menopause, or the end of periods, usually occurs in women between the ages of forty-five and fifty-five. It is a cycle of change, a time for reflection on life and a reassessment of lifestyle. It is an exciting time and doesn't have to be painful or negative, as so much of the media hype would have us believe. In fact, many women feel elated at this stage of their lives, because they find that menopause represents time for them and their needs. It's a time when you can look forward to meeting new people and setting new goals, such as studying a language, enrolling in a university course or even a cooking class. Set goals to be healthier and wiser, and you'll be amazed at how your body will feel. Use prescription medication sparingly, only if you need it and only when you have tried all other avenues.

When your periods stop completely, your doctor should arrange a bone scan to measure your bone density. You should also have a cholesterol test and a cardiovascular check, including a blood pressure reading. If you have a history of breast cancer in the family, it is usually advised not to take any forms of hormone replacement therapy (HRT) for the symptoms of menopause. This is often when women approach their naturopath for help in relieving symptoms.

Menopausal symptoms can appear early, even while regular periods continue. This is often referred to as a pre-menopausal stage and can be treated very well with natural medicine. Symptoms can include anxiety, mild depression, hot flushes, urinary problems, painful intercourse, dry skin and vagina, loss of vitality, confusion and memory lapses.

A blood test can reveal a hormonal imbalance, although sometimes it will return a normal result even though you may be experiencing uncomfortable symptoms. Most doctors will not treat the pre-menopausal stage with hormones and will advise you to include certain foods in your diet and supplement it with natural medicine. If you experience depression at this stage, I recommend you try natural therapies before resorting to stronger medication. I have seen vitamin and herbal supplementation – combined with regular exercise and a healthy diet – work very well in pre-menopausal women.

Periods stop due to the loss of ovary function and a decline of oestrogen and progesterone. When this happens and you have had no periods for six months, symptoms can become more intense, although this is certainly not the case for all women. Even after periods stop, the body continues to make small amounts of hormones from the adrenal glands while it is adjusting to the chemical changes. Women can do so many things to help themselves feel more balanced and healthy, allowing this transition stage to be easier and eliminating much of the negativity that often surrounds hormonal changes.

RECOMMENDATIONS for dealing with menopause

- Foods with a soya bean base can help ease hot flushes and other mild symptoms. Add soya beans or tofu to salads two to three times a week.

- Flaxseed contains high levels of substances known as lignan phytoestrogens, soluble fibre and linoleic acid, which help omega-3 and -6 fatty acids protect against heart disease, so add flaxseed oil to your diet.

- Sage tea is traditionally well known to lift the spirits, so if you are feeling melancholy, drink two to three cups a day.

- Take one vitamin E tablet (250 IU or 500 IU if you do not have high blood pressure) a day to act as an antioxidant, help prevent dry skin and improve circulation.

- Take one fish oil capsule and one evening primrose oil capsule twice daily.

- Take one to two black cohosh tablets daily or as prescribed by your naturopath or doctor, if you are having mood swings.

- Take one vitamin B-complex tablet (containing 50 mg each of the Bs) daily for extra vitality.

- Take one calcium supplement (1000 mg) a day to help keep bones strong.

- Drink two cups of petal tea a day.

- For depression, try two to three St John's wort tablets a day and one magnesium tablet (500 mg) two to three times a day (check with your doctor if you are on other medication).

- Vaginal dryness can be treated with a cream made from a base of vitamin E with 10 ml of calendula oil, 10 ml of evening primrose oil and 20 ml of olive oil. This can be applied morning and evening.

- For insomnia in menopause, take one tablet (3 mg) of melatonin before bed. Menopausal women have been found to have low levels of this hormone, which is vital for deep sleep and has recently been found to have anti-cancer effects.

A tonic for dealing with menopause

Combine equal parts of black cohosh, liquorice, chasteberry, motherwort, chamomile, wild yam, sage and red clover. Take 1 teaspoon two to three times a day to relieve many of the uncomfortable pre-menopausal symptoms.

Will HRT assist me?

Natural medicine can be beneficial on its own or in conjunction with prescribed medicines. You can only decide whether or not to take HRT when you have all the facts. The first consideration is your general health. If there is no breast cancer or osteoporosis in your family history and you have a strong cardiovascular system, you may not wish to take HRT. Similarly, if you have osteoporosis or there is a history of heart disease or breast cancer in your family, it might be preferable to try natural medicine instead of HRT. However, if the symptoms are severe and natural medicine is not working strongly enough, HRT can be a great relief. Bear in mind, though, that recent research recommends that HRT not be taken for more than two years.

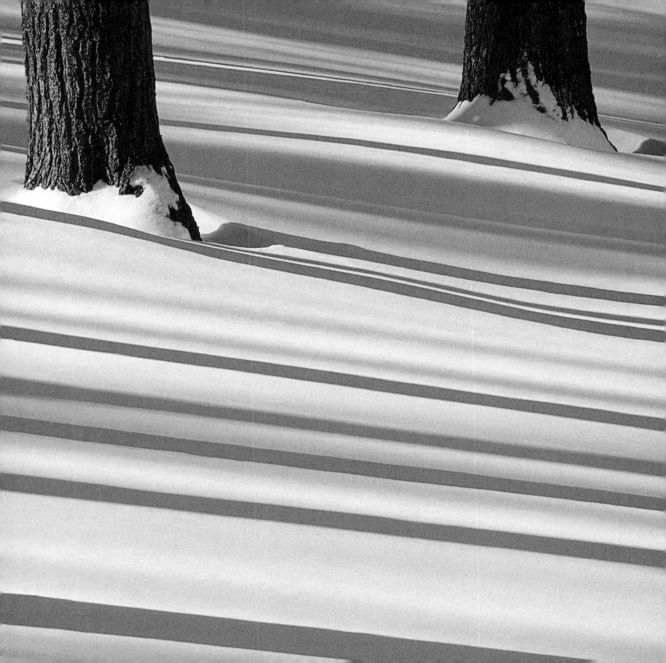

BLACK COHOSH (CIMICIFUGA RACEMOSA)

The root of this native North American plant has been used in the treatment of female reproductive disorders as well as rheumatism and myalgia. Since 1950 it has also been used to treat menopausal symptoms and menstrual disturbances in young women (particularly amenorrhoea). During menopause the LH hormone surges and causes hot flushes; recent research has shown that black cohosh suppresses the LH, providing relief. In trials in Germany, women reported a significant improvement in menopausal symptoms including hot flushes, sweating, insomnia, nervousness and irritability. Black cohosh can be used instead of HRT and can also help women wean off HRT. It can be prescribed by your health practitioner or doctor.

Sex drive

Libido is governed by well-balanced hormones and a healthy diet. Of course, a happy relationship is also important, as is managing stress in your life. Testosterone is a hormone that is generally only associated with men, and many women are unaware that they have small amounts of this hormone too. Some women do not produce enough testosterone, which directly affects their sex drive, during and after menopause. A healthy diet, exercise and restful sleep are vital to a woman's sexual response.

TRIBULUS TERRESTRIS

Tribulus terrestris is a herb that has been shown to enhance testosterone production, which can increase sex drive.

Post-menopause

Menopause can last for six months or for two to three years. Generally you know that it is finished when you feel back to your old self: no more hot flushes, no unusual anxiety, your hope in life is restored and you have a positive outlook. When you feel an improvement, I recommend you stay on your vitamins, cutting down the dosages as you feel better. If symptoms reappear, return to your former vitamin and herbal program.

RECOMMENDATIONS for post-menopause

- Take one to two antioxidant tablets a day for continued wellbeing and to help prevent cancer.
- Take vitamin E (250 IU or 500 IU if you do not have high blood pressure) daily.
- Take two fish oil capsules a day to keep cholesterol under control.
- Take 500 mg calcium each day with 200 mg of magnesium.
- Take one co-enzyme Q10 tablet (60 mg) daily to restore energy and heart integrity.
- If your memory is failing, take a ginkgo tablet once or twice a day, but not in the evenings, because it will keep you awake.

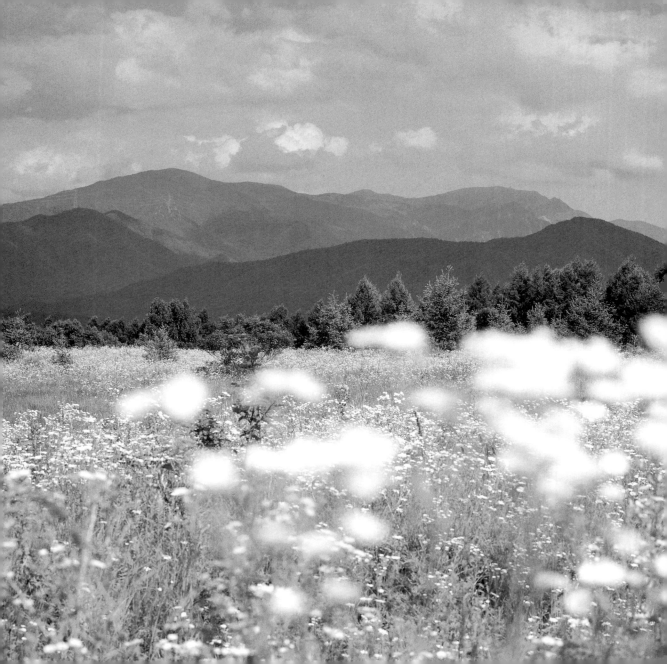

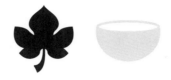

8. Tips for travel

It is always best to prepare your body before long-distance travel. Food, immunity, stress and recovery are important factors to address.

RECOMMENDATIONS before travel

- Try to get eight hours' sleep each night for at least three nights before you travel.

- Take one melatonin tablet (1–3 mg) two to three nights before you travel to prepare your body for a different time zone.

- Take the following supplements for a week prior to flying, to keep your blood thin and help avoid blood clots on the plane: two evening primrose oil capsules a day, vitamin E (250 IU) once a day and B_6 (100 mg) once a day if you suffer from fluid retention.

RECOMMENDATIONS for the plane

- Do not eat junk food. Pre-order vegetarian meals or fruits, because they are lighter on the digestion.

- Drink lots of water to prevent dehydration.

- Avoid alcohol, because it is very dehydrating. If you decide to drink alcohol on the plane, stick to a spirit mixed with soda or tonic water and drink two glasses of water for every glass of alcohol.

- Stretch and move about every few hours to aid circulation, and make sure that while you are sitting you do the foot exercises encouraged by the airlines to prevent blood clots.

- Airlines usually keep eucalyptus and peppermint inhalants on board, which help blocked sinuses and your respiratory system, so ask for these if you feel blocked, especially when landing.

- You can take along a Vicks inhalant and use it to help equalise the pressure in your airways, and so prevent pain and ear problems.

- Try to sleep on the plane; a melatonin tablet or a herbal combination of valerian, passionflower, calcium and vervain may help.

- Do not wear make-up when flying; this will allow your skin to breathe. Use a rich night moisturiser on your face and hands to prevent your skin drying out.

- Take as little as possible on the plane with you. Remember, you have to carry it and a heavy load can add to the fatigue and frustration of jet lag.

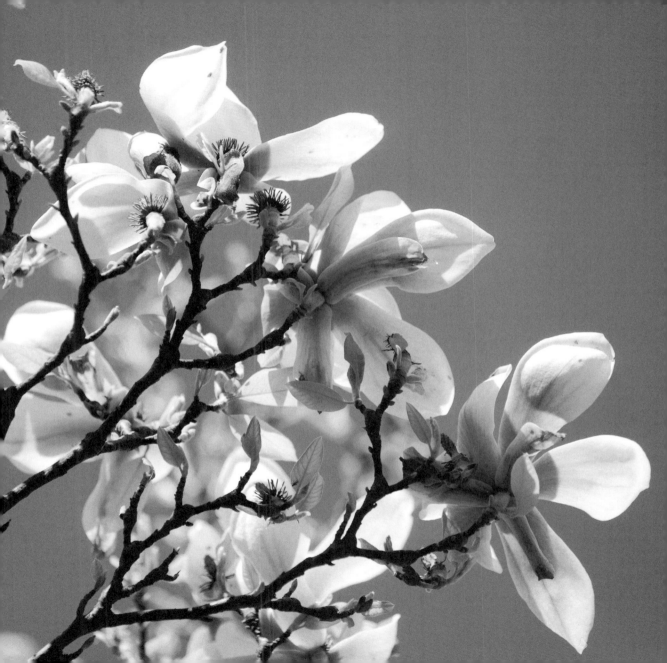

- Take a good book – preferably one you have started to read before the trip and can't put down. So many people quickly buy a new book at the airport and don't like their choice once they begin reading.

- Try to relax and enjoy the trip, whether it is for business or a holiday.

RECOMMENDATIONS for your arrival

If you are going straight to bed when you arrive at your destination, follow these steps.

- Take a long, hot bath, preferably with a cup of Epsom salts added, which will help you sleep. Adding 6–8 drops of lavender oil will also help you relax.

- Stretch for ten minutes before bed.

- Take a melatonin tablet (not more than 3 mg) ten minutes before bed. Continue one tablet a day for three to four days to help your body adjust its time clock. (You may take it for longer – seven to ten days – if you like.)

- If you do not like taking melatonin, take two valerian tablets and one calcium tablet (500–1000 mg) to help you sleep.

- Drink a cup of loose-leaf organic chamomile tea.

- If you haven't eaten properly on the plane and are hungry, have a simple vegetable soup (no spices). Avoid bread, cheese, black tea, coffee or green tea, because these may keep you awake.

- You may wish to watch television to help you relax, but avoid anything violent or the news; choose instead a gentle program or listen to some classical music.

RECOMMENDATIONS for while you are away

These will keep your energy levels high and your immune system healthy, as well as help relieve jet lag.

- Take one antioxidant tablet (60–100 mg) a day.

- If your skin is dry and you are travelling to a cold climate, take two evening primrose oil capsules a day.

- Magnesium assists muscles and prevents cramping, so take one to two tablets a day if you are walking a lot, sightseeing or skiing.

- Take one multivitamin tablet containing B vitamins, iron and folic acid a day for energy and to make up for any depletions while travelling.

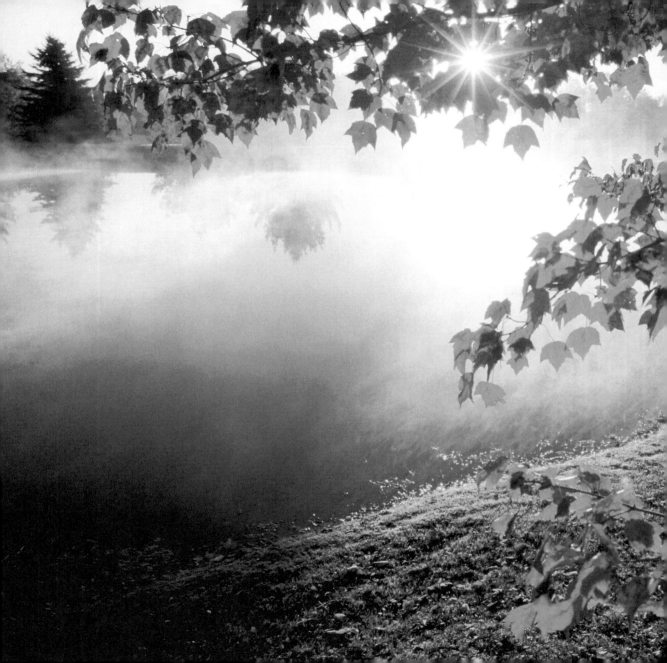

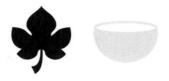

9. Ageing gracefully

We are now living longer than at any time in history. Advances in medical science have played their part in increasing our life spans, but another important factor in our longevity is our increased knowledge of preventative medicine. We look seriously at how exercise, diet, smoking and alcohol affect us and the way we age. On top of that, we can now explore a variety of stimulating work opportunities that were not available to women in the past; these help keep our minds and bodies active.

Combating ageing

This all sounds so overwhelming, and yet the essence of living longer is all to do with our quality of life. Are we happy? Are we active? Do we enjoy good health? Do we use our brains to their full potential? Are we in happy relationships? Do we live in a stimulating environment? Dr David Weeks and Jamie Jones, who researched and wrote a book called *The Super Young*, found in summary three points that made some people appear younger than their counterparts at the same age.

- These people had more energy because they enjoyed quality sleep. During sleep the body repairs the brain, restores depleted substances and repairs damaged cell tissue.

- These people had a stronger resilience to the stresses of life and had the ability to bounce back from disasters in their lives.

- These people had the capacity to adapt to new situations.

The qualities of energy, resilience and adaptability are not, as this study found, all genetic. People *work* on their health to have more energy, and supplementary vitamins and foods can give you greater 'brain power'. The following can be incorporated in your daily life to obtain, over a period of time, greater energy and sharper mental facilities.

RECOMMENDATIONS for ageing well, in mind and body

- Include antioxidant-rich foods in your diet.

- The brain needs fuel to function properly, so avoid low blood sugar levels by eating three meals a day and protein snacks or fruit in between meals.

- Cut out 80 per cent of your junk food intake, including soft drinks, refined sugars, processed meats and tinned foods.

- Excess alcohol destroys brain cells, so cut down your alcohol consumption.

- Drink eight glasses of pure water daily and include herbal teas to your taste.

- Drink raw juices, which contain enzymes for cell rejuvenation.
- Drink some form of concentrated green juice such as wheat grass juice (one tablespoon a day mixed with carrot juice or water), or spirulina or green barley juice. They are rich in peptides and enzymes, which are essential for the development of the feel-good hormones such as endorphins.
- Exercise regularly – three times a week or more.
- Stretch or do yoga for ten minutes a day to keep your joints and muscles supple.
- Spend time outdoors in fresh air with trees, water or mountains.
- Keep out of the strong rays of the midday sun (they can be cancer-forming and ageing) and always use sunscreen.
- Stress depletes important minerals and vitamin B, so try to keep stress levels down.
- If you can, find a happy work environment.
- Do all you can to get out of an unhappy relationship.
- Spend time with friends of all ages and stay involved with younger people.
- Do not smoke or take recreational drugs; they destroy brain cells.
- Take one to two ginkgo tablets a day (avoid these at night, because they will keep you awake).
- Take one co-enzyme Q10 tablet (60–100 mg) a day, to assist oxygen supply to your cardiovascular system.

- Take selenium: 20–30 mg a day.

- Take one to two fish oil capsules daily; these contain omega-3 and -6 fatty acids for the lubrication of joints and prevention of myelin sheath wear and tear.

- Take 2000 mg of lecithin a day. Lecithin contains choline, which protects and restores dendrites in the brain, essential for memory and sharp thinking. It was found in one study that patients with memory loss experienced up to 50 per cent improvement just from choline supplementation. Foods high in lecithin are egg yolks, soya beans, wheat germ and whole wheat products.

Antioxidants

We hear about antioxidants through the media and in health books, but very few people really know what antioxidants are or how they work. To put it simply, free radicals – which are created within the body through normal living and through some external factors – cause oxidation, which can break down cells in the body. Antioxidants are naturally occurring substances that work against the process of oxidation.

Major factors in our modern lifestyle have a profound effect on free radical production, including pollution, refined fatty foods, stress, smoking, recreational drugs and viruses. The breakdown of healthy tissue can lead to cancers, heart disease, chronic bowel problems and numerous other illnesses prevalent in the twenty-first century.

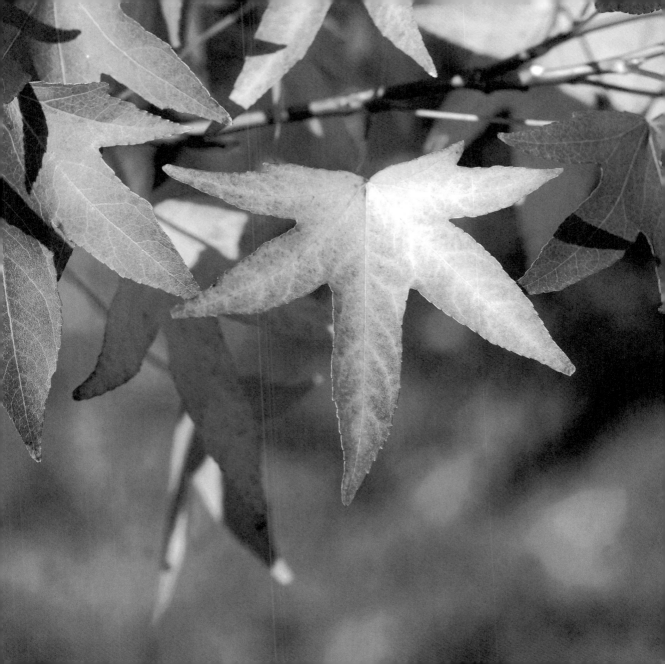

By taking antioxidants regularly through food and vitamin supplements we can slow free radical damage. Antioxidants are an essential part of daily living and not only increase our life span but also improve the quality of our life through greater wellbeing and vitality. The main foods rich in antioxidants are orange fruits and vegetables such as oranges, sweet potato, pumpkin, carrots, mangoes, peaches, paw paw, nectarines and apricots, which contain vitamins C and A. Vitamin E, found in avocados and wheatgerm oils, and in smaller amounts in cold-pressed olive oils and cold-pressed vegetable oils, is also a vital antioxidant. Certain herbs and other food substances, such as garlic, sage, turmeric, rosemary, schisandra and St Mary's thistle, green tea and black tea, grape seed and co-enzyme Q10, have also been found to have significant antioxidant properties.

FISH OILS

Fish oils have been found to protect the myelin sheath, which function with the nerves like the outer plastic coat of an electrical wire. Myelin acts as an insulator and protects the sensitive nerves, helping to conduct impulses. It is thought that those who have keen mental powers in later life may have a genetic predisposition that protects the myelin sheath from breaking down. We would all be wise to take fish oils, ginkgo and antioxidants. Multiple sclerosis sufferers have been found to have inflammation of the myelin sheath, and research is holding out positive hope for more findings on how to restore this sheath in the chronic stages of this illness.

GINKGO (*GINKGO BILOBA*)

The ginkgo is a deciduous tree that has been around for 150 million years. The research of German scientists in the 1960s showed that ginkgo is an excellent treatment for circulation problems. The herb brings more oxygen to the tissues, particularly brain tissue. The leaves contain active substances known as flavonoids. Ginkgo is wonderful for treating problems of memory, tinnitus, dizziness and the effects of high altitude, and it is especially helpful for the early effects of dementia. It can help enhance memory, particularly in the 50-plus age group.

Build happiness/lower stress

High levels of continued stress produce an overabundance of a hormone called cortisol from the adrenal glands. The part of the brain that shuts off this production deteriorates with age. When this happens you react even more strongly to stress and can suffer even more damage to the 'shut-off' mechanism. Research has found that stress is magnified when people feel out of control. It has also been discovered that if you are to reduce your stress levels, you must not allow a problem to build up inside you – if something is worrying you, chat to a friend or family member or see a counsellor.

Brain power boosters

Alertness and memory are key issues for the modern woman who wishes to age gracefully. With this in mind, remember that the brain is an organ that must be exercised daily, so keep up any hobby that engages your mind. Take on new challenges with study, languages, reading and mind games such as puzzles using numbers, words or sentences.

Brain cells do not regenerate, therefore it is vital to preserve what you have and to use natural medicines to assist your memory powers. Scientists have found that three main factors affect longevity and memory loss:

- raised homocystine levels in the blood (this can be tested by your doctor);
- poor circulation and atherosclerosis (hardening of the arteries); and
- inflammation (from arthritis, coeliac disease, irritable bowel, allergies, toxic exposure, alcohol, smoking).

RECOMMENDATIONS to boost brain power

- Folic acid (200–300 mg) can assist in lowering homocystine levels.
- Schisandra (*Schisandra chinensis*) is a Chinese herb known to assist alertness and ease mental fatigue, and is a great detoxifier for the liver. Take one tablet a day.
- Bacopa is a herb used to enhance long-term memory and reduce stress. Take one tablet a day.

- Ginkgo biloba aids short-term memory. Take one tablet a day.

- Exercise regularly to increase oxygen supply to the brain.

- Top 'brain foods' to eat on a daily basis include: broccoli, dark grapes (muscatels), tomatoes, garlic, dark berries, almonds, salmon, carrots and green tea.

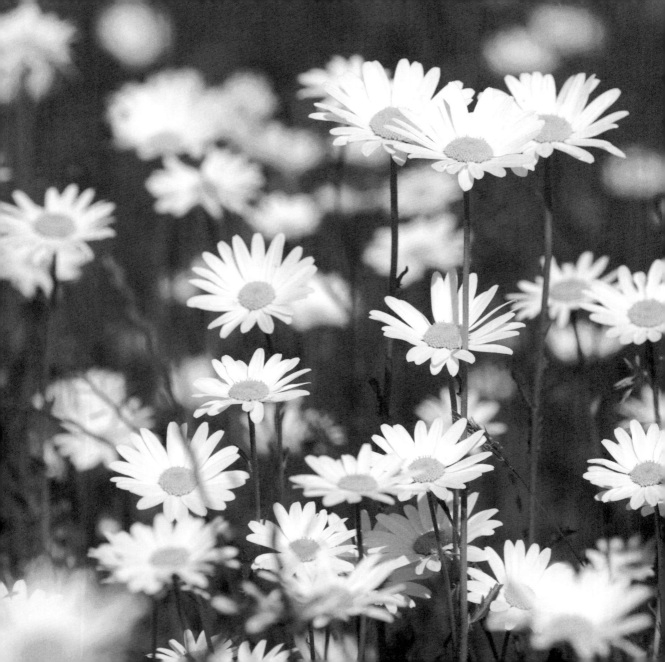

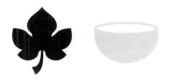

10. Other common female issues

Recurring minor ailments – symptoms can range from thrush to weak nails to a bloated stomach – often indicate an imbalance in the diet. When you improve your eating habits (see Chapter 11, 'Natural Nourishing Recipes', for practical advice and delicious recipes) you will find that most minor issues begin to clear. If you are continually experiencing symptoms that are not related to a more serious condition, it can often be your body telling you that you need to slow down and attend to the small problem before it turns into a larger one.

Sometimes minor symptoms can be hereditary, but there is always a natural way of remedying them before resorting to medication. Preventative action is the key factor in the following issues.

Headaches

Headaches can be a sign of any of the following: hormonal imbalance, a vertebra problem in the neck, muscle tightness in the neck or back, gallstones and kidney stones, constipation, stress, low blood sugar levels or dehydration. If you suffer from headaches it is important that you identify their most likely cause and act to relieve the problem.

RECOMMENDATIONS for easing headaches

- Magnesium helps relax muscle tissue and relieve spasms. Take 400–600 mg a day in powder or tablet form.

- If you have inflammation from an injury, an antioxidant tablet three times a day is essential, with one tablet of bioflavonoids three times a day.

- Feverfew is a herb used in traditional herbal medicine as a preventative and a cure for migraine headaches. You can try taking one tablet three times a day until your headache abates.

Nausea

Nausea can be a sign of several things, including pregnancy, gall bladder problems, an overloaded stomach and poor digestion.

RECOMMENDATIONS for dealing with nausea

- Ginger tablets are marvellous for easing nausea, and are safe to use during pregnancy. Take one after every meal. If gallstones run in your family, ask your doctor for an ultrasound.

- Take one fish oil capsule after each meal (if you don't like the smell or taste of fish oil, try evening primrose oil). These oils assist the gall bladder to eliminate bile, which in turn helps to break down fatty foods in the digestive tract.

Poor kidney function

Our kidneys are vital for excreting waste and reabsorbing any trace minerals and other elements that can be useful. Kidneys have millions of fine tubules, like a very complicated plumbing system, and it is imperative for good health that we keep this tubing clean and drained by taking in fresh liquids each day. If we do not, stagnant waste accumulates in these tubes, causing blockages which can lead to infections such as cystitis, kidney stones and fluid retention.

RECOMMENDATIONS for maintaining healthy kidneys

- Drink eight to ten glasses of filtered water a day, and during and after exercise, to clear the accumulation of wastes and toxins that are released.

- Begin the day with a glass of water at room temperature with the juice of half a lemon added.

- Include a glass of freshly squeezed orange, mango or watermelon juice in your daily intake.

- Include a raw juice of orange and green vegetables daily. Try carrot juice mixed with spinach, wheatgrass and parsley or add 1 teaspoon of spirulina or green barley powder.
- Include fresh homemade soup for a meal or entrée three to four times a week (in summer replace with fresh salads).
- Eat two to three pieces of whole fruit daily.
- Cut out soft drinks, sugar in tea and coffee, excessive amounts of alcohol, cakes and sweet refined snacks.
- Do not smoke.
- Include yoghurt in your diet daily for the good acidophilus bacteria.
- If you have a tendency to cystitis, drink a glass of preservative-free cranberry juice each day.

Cystitis

Mild cystitis is recognised by a feeling of discomfort around the bladder area and the need to urinate frequently. In its severe stages cystitis becomes an infection in the bladder and causes a burning feeling during urination. Before resorting to antibiotics, try natural medicine, which is often very successful. Regular preventative work is essential if you have been suffering these symptoms for a while.

RECOMMENDATIONS for combating cystitis

- Drink eight to ten glasses of water a day.
- Cranberry juice has been found to help a great deal, because it has the ability to slough off the nasty bacteria that cling to the walls of the urinary tract. Drink one to two glasses a day.
- Barley water soothes irritated bladder walls and flushes out any residual infection. Drink three cups a day (use 1 cup of barley to 1 litre of water and simmer for twenty minutes before straining) with the juice of a quarter of a lemon in each glass.
- Echinacea tablets or liquid help fight the infection. Take one tablet or 1 teaspoon of the tincture every four hours.
- Buffered vitamin C (such as Ester C): take 1 teaspoon in water every four hours.
- Garlic tablets: take one every four hours.

A tonic for combating cystitis

Combine equal parts of buchu, uvaursi, echinacea, nettle and cornsilk. Take 1 teaspoon in cranberry juice three to four times a day until you feel better, then once a day for two weeks.

If the cystitis does not improve then you may need an antibiotic. You may still take the natural medicines alongside this, as they will help your immune system. Be aware that cystitis can be an ongoing problem if you do not drink at least eight glasses of water daily.

CRANBERRY 'UNA DE GATO' (*VACCINIUM MACROCARPON*)

Cranberry juice contains procyanidins, which work by stopping bacteria from clinging to the mucosal walls of the urinary tract. For women who have had chronic urinary tract problems, it is vital to include this juice on a regular basis to prevent infections. Always look for the purest form of cranberry juice, because some contain added sugar. Alternatively you can take one tablet twice a day.

Thrush

Thrush shows itself with an annoying white discharge from the vagina and itching. Sometimes thrush can show in the mouth as a white filmy residue on the tongue. It can be exacerbated before and during your period. Thrush is a sign of *Candida albicans*, an overgrowth of the bacterium candida, and often occurs when an overuse of antibiotics destroys much of the bowel's healthy bacteria. Hence eat plenty of yoghurt with acidophilus when taking antibiotics and avoid foods high in sugar, because sugar feeds candida. It is important to note that any bacteria from a bowel motion needs to be wiped away thoroughly from the area between the vagina and the anus.

RECOMMENDATIONS for combating thrush

- Avoid foods that encourage candida, particularly yeasty foods such as bread, wine and beer; fermented cheeses; and refined sugars such as chocolates, sugary desserts, cakes and sweet biscuits.
- Eat yoghurt with added acidophilus daily.
- Make sure you are not constipated, because this breeds more candida.
- Take 1 teaspoon of acidophilus powder (available at health stores) in a glass of water before breakfast and dinner.
- Combine ½ teaspoon of the acidophilus powder with a little water to make a paste and place it in your vagina two to three times a day.
- Garlic has been found to help eliminate thrush, so include garlic in your food as often as possible and take one garlic tablet after each meal until symptoms cease.
- A herb called pau d'arco can help; take 1 teaspoon in half a glass of water twice a day until symptoms cease.

Fibroids and cysts

Fibroids in the uterus or on the ovaries are quite common, and they can occur in women of all ages. Prolonged pain and discomfort in the pelvic area and acne are some symptoms that may indicate you have fibroids or cysts, and an ultrasound can confirm whether you have them and, if you do, how big they are. Check with your doctor to ascertain if they are any threat to your ongoing health. Sometimes they need to be removed surgically if they are large. Generally women feel much better after this procedure, especially without the continual bloating that accompanies fibroids.

Often smaller cysts on the ovaries come and go according to a woman's monthly cycle. Women are often prescribed the contraceptive pill to assist in regulating oestrogen and progesterone, which will reduce the occurrence of cysts.

RECOMMENDATIONS for treating fibroids and cysts

- Vitamin B_6: 200 mg a day helps to dispel minor cysts.
- Magnesium can ease pain: take 100 mg two to three times a day.
- Take chasteberry: one tablet a day for two weeks before your period often takes away many of the minor symptoms and is safe and effective even for adolescents.

Poor circulation and high cholesterol

Hereditary patterns play a major role in problems related to the heart and circulation. The following recommendations are vital if you have a tendency towards high cholesterol and blood pressure, especially if you do not exercise and you smoke, are overweight, have a high alcohol intake and/or eat junk food high in fat and refined products. Studies have found that women who have followed a low-fat diet and included soya beans and greens in their daily diet have lower incidences of heart dis-

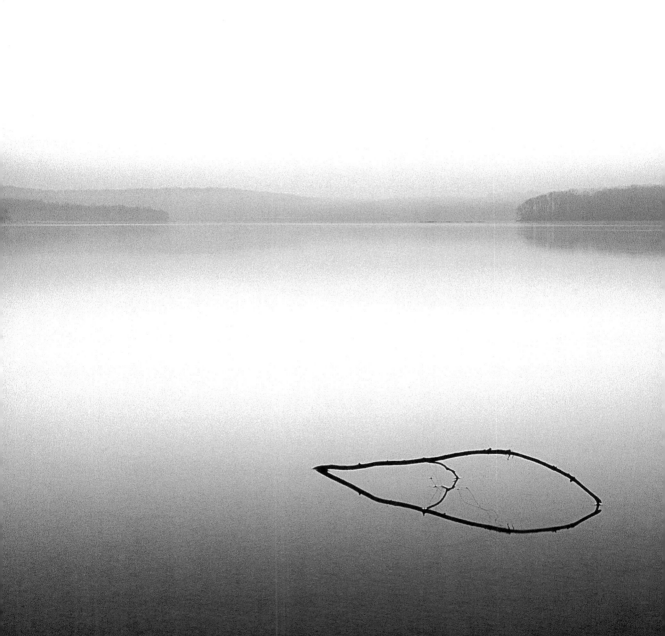

ease and high cholesterol. Many women have high cholesterol when they are going through a hormonal change, and this should be addressed. Check with your doctor to determine your ratio of good and bad cholesterol.

RECOMMENDATIONS for improving circulation and lowering cholesterol

- Eliminate deep-fried foods from your diet and cut right back on saturated fats, including butter, high-fat milk and cream and cheese. Use low-fat substitutes.

- Sauté foods in olive oil or vegetable oil only once a week. It's much better to grill, steam and bake (without fat or oil).

- Limit your chocolate intake. For a sweet treat, try carob, freshly stewed fruits or a muesli bar with grains and dried fruit.

- Drink lots of freshly squeezed citrus fruits such as oranges and lemons, or pineapple juice because they assist in lowering fats.

- Include in your diet avocados and salmon for their omega-3 and -6 fatty acids, which increase the 'good' form of cholesterol. Use cold-pressed oils on salads, but do not use any oil if you have high cholesterol.

- Exercise regularly with some cardio or aerobic work. Ask at your gym for help in determining the level you should be working at and what your heart rate should be. Power walking for an hour each day (five days a week) is ideal.

- Stretch your muscles so your blood can eliminate any fluid gathering in the lower part of your body. Yoga or Pilates is good for this.

- Keep your circulation moving by drinking fresh filtered water in between meals (aim for 1–2 litres a day).

- Undertake a three-day detox (see Chapter 5, 'Detox') each month.

- Take one capsule of salmon oil twice a day.

- Take 500 IU of vitamin E a day.

- Try dandelion coffee instead of normal coffee. Roasted dandelion root is delicious as a coffee substitute.

- Cut back on alcohol; try to stick to one or two glasses of red wine three times a week.

A tonic to improve circulation and lower cholesterol

Combine equal parts of St Mary's thistle, dandelion, hawthorn berry, schisandra and ginger. Take 1 teaspoon twice a day in water or juice.

High blood pressure

If you follow the advice for improving circulation and lowering cholesterol, you will lose weight, which is a must for anyone who is overweight and has cardiovascular problems. The following recommendations are beneficial if you are in the early stages of developing high blood pressure or you are prone to high blood pressure. You must also try to reduce your stress levels.

RECOMMENDATIONS for avoiding high blood pressure

- Take low-dose vitamin E tablets: 100–200 IU daily (check with your doctor).

- Caffeine raises blood pressure, so avoid caffeine in tea, coffee and green tea.

- Take one antioxidant tablet which includes vitamins A, C and E each day (check with your doctor).

- One co-enzyme Q10 tablet (30–60 mg a day) is vital for any heart problem.

- Take fish oil: one capsule after breakfast and one after dinner.

- Meditation can assist in lowering blood pressure.

- Hawthorn berry is a herb that assists normal heart function and can be taken whether you have high or low blood pressure; it also helps fluid retention around the ankles: take one tablet after each meal.

- Take one garlic tablet in the morning and one at night each day.

Varicose veins and broken capillaries

Saline injections and laser treatment can treat fine broken capillaries, but the following recommendations may clear the veins and prevent broken capillaries from spreading.

RECOMMENDATIONS for treating varicose veins and broken capillaries

- Take one bioflavonoid tablet (500 mg) with vitamin C (1000–2000 mg) for absorption, three times a day to strengthen the fine vein walls.

- Drink freshly squeezed orange juice, including the pithy part that contains the bioflavonoids, as well as pineapple juice and fruits rich in vitamin A, including mangoes, apricots, peaches and papaya; these all strengthen vein walls.

- Take one horse chestnut herb tablet after each meal.

- Vitamin E is the number-one antioxidant for veins; take 200–600 IU daily.

- Sleep with a pillow under your feet to assist blood flow, and keep your feet elevated as often as possible.

HORSE CHESTNUT (*AESCULUS HIPPOCASTANUM*)

This is a wonderful herb for treating varicose veins, especially if there is oedema (swelling) of the feet or legs. (It doesn't help fine broken capillaries on the face.) Horse chestnut works very well in elderly patients and if you are prone to thrombosis after surgery. It can also be used as a preventative for blood clotting when you are flying. Take 1–3 tablets (200 mg) of a 5:1 concentrate each day.

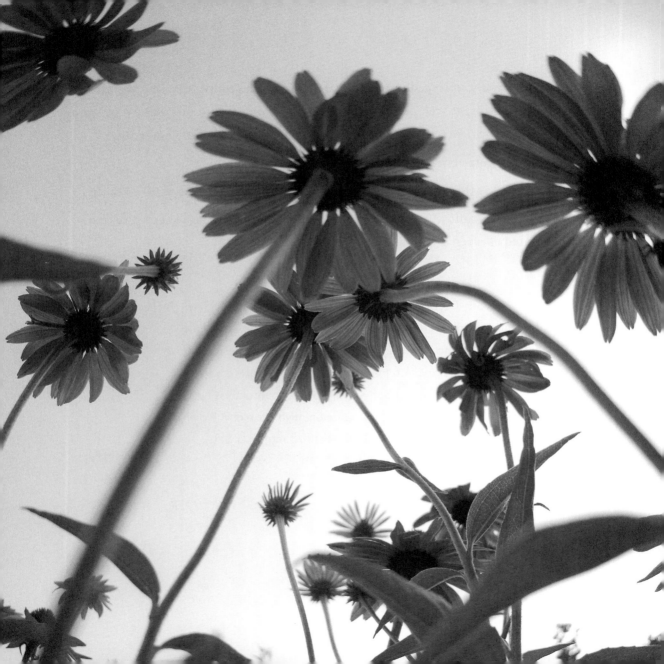

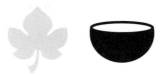

11. Natural nourishing recipes

The recipes in this chapter focus on simple, healthy eating, with dishes you can prepare in a short time with the minimum of fuss, according to your individual health needs. I have used foods that are nourishing in every way – foods that make you feel good and give you energy to get you through each day. When we consume good quality protein, fruit, vegetables, grains, salads, nuts, seeds, water, herbal teas and raw juices, combine them with small amounts of fats, and throw herbs and spices in to enhance the flavours, we are feeding and nourishing every cell of our bodies.

It really is easy to learn these basics and create a range of interesting, nourishing and delicious food for yourself and your family. With these recipes you can prepare a home-cooked meal in a short time, and feel the benefits of natural flavours, have more time with your family and save money on takeaway and restaurant food.

It is important to be creative and flexible in your cooking. If, for example, I have suggested vegetables you don't like, simply exchange them for others of the same colour. I have included recipes for red and white meat, but many of the other dishes are suitable for vegetarians. You don't have to go out and buy exotic ingredients, because taking care of yourself and eating well should be inexpensive and easy. It's about lifestyle and balance.

See the following guide to find the recipes suitable to your health needs.

Quick reference guide to healthy cooking
Use this guide to find the recipes suitable to your health needs.

Anaemia (low iron)

Angela's spinach and cheese bake   *p 180*

Beetroot and asparagus salad   *p 152*

Butter bean, potato and spinach salad   *p 150*

Carrot and beetroot juice   *p 115*

Carrot, spinach and beet greens juice   *p 117*

Cherry juice   *p 122*

Jamie's osso bucco with parsnip mash   *p 186*

Jamie's Thai beef salad   *p 190*

Lamb and lentils on a bed
   of mashed potato   *p 204*

Lamb casserole   *p 212*

Mixed salad with nuts   *p 142*

Muscat grape juice   *p 120*

Spinach and rice   *p 184*

Arthritis

Avocado, mint and pea salad   *p 141*

Baked apples and pears   *p 217*

Barramundi, lemon and potato   *p 188*

Butter bean rissoles   *p 203*

Carrot and celery juice   *p 115*

Carrot and ginger juice   *p 116*

Carrot, beetroot and ginger juice   *p 116*

Cherry juice   *p 122*

Couscous salad   *p 146*

Fish with soy sauce and ginger   *p 200*

Jamie's whole sardines with roasted garlic,
   olive and fennel salad   *p 144*

Kingfish with fresh mint sauce   *p 213*

Maria's peasant-style chicken with
   rosemary   *p 182*

Minestrone soup   *p 157*

Arthritis (cont . . .)

Pan-fried salmon   *p 179*
Poached pears   *p 215*
Rice salad   *p 138*

Stone fruit salad   *p 128*
Whole baked snapper   *p 193*

Asthma

Beetroot and asparagus salad   *p 152*
Buckwheat pancakes   *p 129*
Butter bean rissoles   *p 203*
Carrot and ginger juice   *p 116*
Chicken and vegetable casserole   *p 185*
Citrus fruit salad   *p 128*
Jamie's whole sardines with roasted garlic,
    olive and fennel salad   *p 144*
Kingfish with fresh mint sauce   *p 213*
Lamb and lentils on a bed
    of mashed potato   *p 204*

Lamb casserole   *p 212*
Peach, apricot and mango juice   *p 121*
Poached pears   *p 215*
Rice salad   *p 138*
Salmon rice rissoles   *p 206*
Stone fruit salad   *p 128*
Summer Delight tea   *p 127*
Tofu and shiitake mushroom
    stir-fry   *p 194*
Whole baked snapper   *p 193*

Cholesterol

Apple juice   *p 122*
Avocado, mint and pea salad   *p 141*
Barramundi, lemon and potato   *p 188*
Butter bean, potato and spinach
    salad   *p 150*
Carrot and celery juice   *p 115*
Cauliflower and broccoli soup   *p 156*
Chickpea and avocado salad   *p 151*
Citrus fruit salad   *p 128*
Energy porridge   *p 134*
Fish with soy sauce and ginger   *p 200*

Homemade muesli   *p 133*
Jamie's whole sardines with roasted garlic,
    olive and fennel salad   *p 144*
Kingfish with fresh mint sauce   *p 213*
Oatmeal porridge   *p 133*
Pan-fried salmon   *p 179*
Pearl perch with Corn Flakes crusty
    coating   *p 211*
Rice salad   *p 138*
Salmon rice rissoles   *p 206*
Whole baked snapper   *p 193*

Circulation

Beetroot and asparagus salad   *p 152*
Carrot, beetroot and ginger juice   *p 116*
Citrus fruit salad   *p 128*
Fish with soy sauce and ginger   *p 200*
Kingfish with fresh mint sauce   *p 213*
Lamb and lentils on a bed
   of mashed potato   *p 204*

Maria's peasant-style chicken with
   rosemary   *p 182*
Prawns with Asian herbs   *p 205*
Scrambled curried eggs   *p 135*
Spaghetti with garlic, oil and chilli   *p 192*

Concentration

Buckwheat pancakes   *p 129*
Butter bean, potato and spinach
   salad   *p 150*
Carrot, beetroot and ginger juice   *p 116*
Chickpea and avocado salad   *p 151*
Egg and asparagus salad   *p 143*
Energy porridge   *p 134*
Fish with soy sauce and ginger   *p 200*
The healthy omelette   *p 136*
Jamie's lentil and bacon salad   *p 140*
Jamie's osso bucco with parsnip mash   *p 186*
Kingfish with fresh mint sauce   *p 213*

Maria's peasant-style chicken with
   rosemary   *p 182*
Muscat grape juice   *p 120*
Oatmeal porridge   *p 133*
Pan-fried salmon   *p 179*
Peach, apricot and mango juice   *p 121*
Rice salad   *p 138*
Salmon rice rissoles   *p 206*
Spinach and rice   *p 184*
Stone fruit salad   *p 128*
Tuna macaroni   *p 183*
Whole baked snapper   *p 193*

Depression and irritability

Anzac biscuits   *p 216*
Apres tea   *p 125*
Baked sweet bananas with cinnamon   *p 219*
Barramundi, lemon and potato   *p 188*
Couscous salad   *p 146*
Energy porridge   *p 134*

Fish with soy sauce and ginger   *p 200*
Homemade muesli   *p 133*
Jamie's osso bucco with parsnip mash   *p 186*
Jamie's Thai beef salad   *p 190*
Jamie's whole sardines with roasted garlic,
   olive and fennel salad   *p 144*

Depression and irritability (cont . . .)

Kebabs   *p 196*

Kingfish with fresh mint sauce   *p 213*

Minestrone soup   *p 157*

My favourite Niçoise salad   *p 139*

Oatmeal porridge   *p 133*

Orange and lemon juice   *p 119*

Pan-fried salmon   *p 179*

Peach, apricot and mango juice   *p 121*

Pearl perch with Corn Flakes crusty
coating   *p 212*

Roast spatchcock   *p 198*

Soy chicken and potatoes   *p 209*

Spaghetti vongole   *p 208*

Spinach and rice   *p 184*

Vegetable rissoles   *p 200*

Watermelon juice   *p 124*

Detox/liver

Avocado, mint and pea salad   *p 141*

Beetroot and asparagus salad   *p 152*

Carrot and beetroot juice   *p 115*

Carrot and sultana salad   *p 137*

Carrot, cabbage and turmeric juice   *p 118*

Cauliflower and broccoli soup   *p 156*

Chicken and vegetable casserole   *p 185*

Chickpea and avocado salad   *p 151*

Cleansing noodle soup   *p 158*

Kebabs   *p 196*

Kingfish with fresh mint sauce   *p 213*

Lemon Tang tea   *p 126*

Mixed salad with nuts   *p 142*

Mulberry, blackberry, raspberry and
cranberry juice   *p 123*

Muscat grape juice   *p 120*

Peach, apricot and mango juice   *p 121*

Pearl perch with Corn Flakes crusty
coating   *p 211*

Triple E tea   *p 127*

Vegetable rissoles   *p 200*

Whole baked snapper   *p 193*

Digestive problems/ulcers/heartburn

Apple juice   *p 122*

Apres tea   *p 125*

Apricot coconut balls   *p 215*

Avocado, mint and pea salad   *p 141*

Baked apples and pears   *p 218*

Baked sweet bananas with cinnamon   *p 219*

Barley soup   *p 154*

Buckwheat pancakes   *p 129*

Butterfly zucchini pasta   *p 192*

Carrot and sultana salad   *p 137*

Carrot, cabbage and turmeric juice   *p 118*

Couscous salad   *p 146*

Digestive problems/ulcers/heartburn (cont . . .)

Energy

Fluid retention/sluggish kidneys/kidney stones

Barley soup   *p 155*
Beetroot and asparagus salad   *p 152*
Carrot and celery juice   *p 115*
Carrot, celery and parsley juice   *p 117*
Kingfish with fresh mint sauce   *p 213*
Lemon Tang tea   *p 126*

Mulberry, blackberry, raspberry and
   cranberry juice   *p 123*
Pan-fried salmon   *p 179*
Poached pears   *p 215*
Watermelon juice   *p 124*
Whole baked snapper   *p 193*

Gluten-free

Buckwheat pancakes   *p 129*
Maria's peasant-style chicken with
   rosemary   *p 182*
Pan-fried salmon   *p 179*

Rice salad   *p 138*
Spinach and rice   *p 184*
Whole baked snapper   *p 193*

Hypoglycaemia (low blood sugar)

Angela's spinach and cheese bake   *p 180*
Anzac biscuits   *p 216*
Buckwheat pancakes   *p 129*
Butter bean, potato and spinach salad   *p 150*
Butter bean rissoles   *p 203*
Cheese, tomato and basil pizza   *p 168*
Cherry juice   *p 122*
Chicken and vegetable casserole   *p 185*
Chicken drumsticks   *p 201*
Chickpea and avocado salad   *p 151*
Chickpea spread   *p 163*
Couscous salad   *p 146*
Energy porridge   *p 134*
The healthy omelette   *p 136*
Homemade muesli   *p 133*

Jamie's lentil and bacon salad   *p 140*
Jamie's osso bucco with parsnip mash   *p 186*
Jamie's Thai beef salad   *p 190*
Jamie's whole sardines with roasted garlic,
   olive and fennel salad   *p 144*
Kebabs   *p 195*
Lamb and lentils on a bed of mashed
   potato   *p 204*
Lamb casserole   *p 212*
Maria's peasant-style chicken with
   rosemary   *p 182*
Mixed salad with nuts   *p 142*
Mulberry, blackberry, raspberry and
   cranberry juice   *p 123*
My favourite antipasto platter   *p 169*

Hypoglycaemia (low blood sugar) (cont . . .)

Immune system (coughs, colds, flus)

Insomnia

Irritable bowel

Irritable bowel (cont . . .)

Libido

PMT

PMT (cont . . .)

Pumpkin and sage pasta *p 208*

Rice salad *p 138*

Roast spatchcock *p 196*

Tofu and shiitake mushroom stir-fry *p 194*

Tuna macaroni *p 183*

Watermelon juice *p 124*

Rheumatism (muscle pain)

Baked apples and pears *p 217*

Barramundi, lemon and potato *p 188*

Butter bean rissoles *p 203*

Butterfly zucchini pasta *p 189*

Carrot and celery juice *p 115*

Cherry juice *p 122*

Chicken and vegetable casserole *p 185*

Couscous salad *p 146*

Fish with soy sauce and ginger *p 200*

Jamie's whole sardines with roasted garlic,

olive and fennel salad *p 144*

Kingfish with fresh mint sauce *p 213*

Maria's peasant-style chicken with rosemary *p 182*

Minestrone soup *p 157*

Pearl perch with Corn Flakes crusty coating *p 211*

Poached pears *p 215*

Rice salad *p 138*

Stone fruit salad *p 128*

Skin – acne

Barramundi, lemon and potato *p 188*

Carrot and beetroot juice *p 115*

Carrot, spinach and beet greens juice *p 117*

Chickpea and avocado salad *p 151*

Couscous salad *p 146*

Kingfish with fresh mint sauce *p 213*

Minestrone soup *p 157*

Peach, apricot and mango juice *p 121*

Vegetable rissoles *p 198*

Whole baked snapper *p 193*

Skin – dry

Avocado, mint and pea salad *p 141*

Baked apples and pears *p 217*

Barramundi, lemon and potato *p 188*

Carrot, spinach and beet greens juice *p 117*

Minestrone soup *p 157*

Mixed salad with nuts *p 142*

Pan-fried salmon *p 179*

Peach, apricot and mango juice *p 121*

Pearl perch with Corn Flakes crusty coating *p 211*

Skin – dry (cont . . .)

Sports energy

Vegetarian

Wheat- and yeast-free

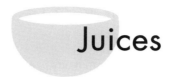

Juices

Carrot and celery   makes 250 ml

This juice eases arthritis and sore joints. Celery juice is high in natural sodium to assist joint mobility.

2½ medium carrots, trimmed and washed
1¼ sticks of celery, washed

Process ingredients in an electric juicer and serve.

Carrot and beetroot   makes 250 ml

This juice helps fight acne and dermatitis. The carrot juice detoxifies the liver; the beetroot juice cleanses the spleen, which is helpful for vibrant skin.

3½ medium carrots, trimmed and washed
1 small wedge of beetroot (approximately 25 g), washed

Process ingredients in an electric juicer and serve.

Carrot and ginger   makes 250 ml

This juice soothes constipation. The carrot juice stimulates liver enzymes and cleans a sluggish liver, stimulating cleansing of the bowel; the ginger increases circulation and brings heat and life to a slow bowel and sore joints.

4 medium carrots, trimmed and washed
small knob of fresh ginger (approximately 10 g), peeled

Process ingredients in an electric juicer and serve.

Carrot, beetroot and ginger   makes 250 ml

This juice is wonderful for those with arthritis or cold hands and feet. The ginger assists circulation to external joints; the carrot juice and beetroot juice clear the liver, allowing fewer free radicals to accumulate in the joints.

3–4 medium carrots, trimmed and washed
1 small wedge of beetroot (approximately 25 g)
3 knobs ginger (approximately 30 g), peeled

Process ingredients in an electric juicer and serve.

Carrot, spinach and beet greens   makes 250 ml

*This juice is ideal for anaemia sufferers and for women as a pep-up before periods.
The spinach contains high amounts of chlorophyll, folic acid and iron. For women
who do not absorb iron well, drink this juice daily or until your iron levels are normal,
then drink it twice a week.*

1½ medium carrots, trimmed and washed
½ bunch English spinach, washed
5–6 beetroot stems and leaves, washed

Process ingredients in an electric juicer and serve.

Carrot, celery and parsley   makes 250 ml

*This juice eases fluid retention. Celery is a wonderful, safe diuretic, particularly for
fluid retention associated with diseases and also before a period. Parsley is a strong
herb and is high in folic acid; use a small amount, because it can be a powerful
cleanser of the kidneys.*

2 large carrots, trimmed and washed
2 sticks celery
6 sprigs parsley, washed

Process ingredients in an electric juicer and serve.

Carrot, cabbage and turmeric   makes 250 ml

This juice is ideal for people with ulcers, irritable bowel syndrome, cancer or varicose veins. The cabbage juice contains an amazing vitamin called vitamin U, which has a wonderful history of healing all forms of ulcers and inflamed mucous membranes. (Research is continuing regarding the benefits of cabbage as an anti-cancer agent.) Turmeric is a great antioxidant for heart disease, cancer, arthritis and any liver disease. This formula is an excellent way to destroy parasites in the bowel. (If you are not used to the taste of cabbage juice, sip on this formula slowly so your digestion can adapt. Add 1 clove of garlic for added antibacterial effect – especially useful to fight against parasites in the bowel.)

1½ medium carrots, trimmed and washed

⅛ of medium cabbage (approximately 285 g), washed and shredded

1 knob fresh turmeric (or ½ teaspoon powder)

Process ingredients in an electric juicer and serve.

Orange and lemon   makes 250 ml

This juice fights colds, flus and bronchial problems. All orange fruits (and vegetables) are high in antioxidants, which work against a sluggish liver and major diseases such as cancer and cardiovascular disease. Orange juice is very high in vitamin C; the whole pith put back in the juice holds the bioflavonoids, which are a natural anti-inflammatory for sinus passages. Lemon juice is great for cleansing the body of mucus, and it also stimulates the digestive juices, particularly in the liver and pancreas.

If you are very 'fluey', add 1 teaspoon chopped fresh ginger to this juice. If the juice upsets your digestion, alternate slow sips of this juice with a glass of water with honey added. This last option is excellent if you have a flu-related fever.

2½ medium oranges, peeled leaving a little of the pith, chopped and seeds removed
1 small lemon, peeled leaving a little of the pith, chopped and seeds removed

Process ingredients in an electric juicer and serve.

Orange, pineapple, lemon and grapefruit   makes 250 ml

This juice eases sinus problems and arthritis. Although an acidic fruit, pineapple contains high amounts of a bioflavonoid called bromelain, which can assist joint pain and soothe inflamed sinus passages. The orange juice assists liver function.

½ medium orange, peeled leaving a little of the pith, chopped and seeds removed
200 g pineapple, skin removed and cored
½ small lemon, peeled leaving a little of the pith, chopped and seeds removed
½ medium grapefruit, peeled leaving a little of the pith, chopped and seeds removed

Process ingredients in an electric juicer and serve.

Muscat grape   makes 250 ml

This is a great blood cleanser and is excellent as part of a detox program. Although high in sugar, muscat grapes are also high in flavonoids (antioxidants that fight against cancer) and vitamin C. If you have hypoglycaemia, dilute the juice with water (50 per cent juice, 50 per cent water) . This juice is wonderful for children who are anaemic or do not like eating green vegetables.

2–3 cups of muscat grapes, washed and stems removed

Process grapes in an electric juicer and serve.

Peach, apricot and mango   makes 250 ml

This juice provides an antioxidant liver boost for the skin and aids digestion. All these fruits are from the 'stone' family and aid digestion. They are high in the orange-coloured flavonoids called caratenoids that scavenge free radicals in the body, particularly in the liver. This juice is wonderful for those who need a very alkaline effect on the blood, or who suffer from heartburn, irritable bowel or acne.

175 g peaches, stones removed
200 g apricots, stones removed
200 g firm mango, peeled and stone removed

Process ingredients in an electric juicer and serve.

Strawberry, kiwifruit and white grape   makes 250 ml

This juice enhances the immune system to fight bronchitis, flus and colds. These 'little seed' fruits can be acidic to those with sensitive skin, but they are very high in vitamin C. Drink 1 glass a day before the winter months (at least 3 weeks before).

⅓ cup (approximately 100 g) strawberries, washed and stems removed
⅓ cup (approximately 100 g) kiwifruit, peeled
1 cup white grapes, washed and stems removed

Process ingredients in an electric juicer and serve.

Cherry   makes 250 ml

This juice targets anaemia, gout, arthritis and rheumatism. Cherries are a wonderful fruit with a rich supply of iron for anaemia and joint pain; they clear out the spleen (storage of blood cells) and assist the pancreas (controls sugar levels in blood). You can mix this juice with dark grape juice for children who suffer from anaemia, because the grape juice makes the juice sweeter and adds more antioxidants for growth and good health.

5 cups pitted fresh cherries, washed

Process cherries in an electric juicer and serve.

Apple   makes 250 ml

This juice is beneficial for cigarette smokers and those with indigestion, high cholesterol, toxic exposure to lead and mercury, and cancer. Apples contain pectin, an active ingredient that clears fat from arteries and helps eliminate mercury from lead exposure from the liver, and alleviates free radical damage from chemo- and radiation therapy in cancer patients.

3 medium apples

Process apples in an electric juicer and serve.

Mulberry, blackberry, raspberry and cranberry   makes 250 ml

This juice targets cystitis, kidney problems, a sluggish liver and incontinence. Filled with antioxidants, it is powerful against major diseases, but it can be very sweet, so add water if necessary. This juice is excellent for elderly people who have weak bladders. Berries are also thought to assist vision. If you are unable to find the fresh berries, buy small bottles of organic juice and mix in the same proportions as the recipe.

approximately 1 cup mulberries
approximately 1 cup blackberries
½ cup raspberries
1 cup cranberries

Process ingredients in an electric juicer and serve.

Pear   makes 250 ml

This juice soothes constipation, irritable bowel, coughs and sinus pain. It is gentle as a laxative for irregular bowel motions, and is safe for all ages over three years.

3 medium, firm ripe pears

Process pears in an electric juicer and serve.

Watermelon   makes 250 ml

This juice alleviates fluid retention, irritable bowel and depression. It is a wonderful juice for all ages, and cools the body in summer. You can juice the white rind, which is high in silicon to assist skin, nails and hair. Watermelon juice is also a great diuretic to prevent fluid retention for women before periods.

approximately 400 g watermelon flesh, seeds removed
approximately 10 g watermelon rind

Process ingredients in an electric juicer and serve.

Herbal teas

Herbal teas can play a vital, nourishing role in preventing and treating ailments. As a herbalist and naturopath, I have created a range of organic, loose-leaf, Australian-grown teas that will help you increase your daily fluid intake as well as prevent and soothe common ailments affecting the digestive and nervous systems. Use the following guide to assist your choice. These teas also help carry nutrients around the body and stimulate the excretion of wastes from the blood.

Herbal teas can be used in a number of ways: as a warm tea drink all year round or as iced tea (or even in iceblock form) in summer. Herbal teas are also a great substitute for soft drinks filled with sugar, preservatives and colourings; and you can add honey to sweeten all herbal teas if you or your children have a sweet tooth.

Only buy herbal tea in the organic, loose-leaf form. The tea in herbal tea bags is generally ground down to a powder and has therefore lost the essential oil that is needed for the tea to have a healing effect. They may have a nice taste through added flavourings, but they will not have the therapeutic value required.

- **Apres** is a wonderful after-dinner tea with a delicate chamomile flavour. The tea contains chamomile, fennel, aniseed and peppermint. This tea is suitable for those who suffer from anxiety, stress, poor digestion, heartburn and mild insomnia. Fennel, aniseed and peppermint all benefit those with poor digestion and help to calm an aggravated stomach.

- **Berry** is rich, warm and sweet. It contains hawthorn berries, elder berries and juniper berries. Hawthorn berry assists circulatory problems and has antioxidant properties. Elder and juniper berries assist the sweet taste of this natural herbal tea.

- **Chamomile** is the perfect post-dinner/pre-slumber tea. It soothes the stomach, encourages relaxation and is excellent for PMT, digestive pain, insomnia and children suffering from colic.

- **Green** tea is high in antioxidants for daily health and wellbeing. It contains some caffeine but also has polyphenols, which are a great antioxidant for the lungs and liver. This tea helps control cholesterol and assists in weight loss.

- **Lemon Myrtle** is a unique Australian herb known for its delicate lemon flavour and its healing effects in alleviating colds and flus, and is generally a great tonic if you need a boost.

- **Lemon Tang** contains lemongrass and peppermint. This tea is ideal after fatty meals to help in the digestive process. It is cooling and soothing in hot weather and assists the kidneys, nervous system and liver. It is also very refreshing and soothing for a hangover.

- **Peppermint** tea soothes and refreshes the mind and body. It cleanses the palate, assists the nervous system and aids digestion, especially after fatty food, fish and meat dishes.

- **Petal** tea contains organic red clover, lemongrass, lavender, rose petals and chamomile. This tea assists in cleansing the blood. It also helps those who suffer from stress and anxiety because it relaxes the body, and it is an ideal cleanser for the skin.

- **Summer Delight** contains organic spearmint, peppermint, lemongrass and aniseed. This minty tea is ideal for assisting digestion by stimulating digestive enzymes and relaxing and calming the body. It also helps fight sinus and bronchial problems, is a cleanser for the skin and helps prevent unhealthy bacteria.

- **Triple E** contains liquorice root, aniseed, fennel and peppermint. This tea has a profound healing effect on the bowel and stomach, helping with sluggishness and heartburn. Pure liquorice root works as a mild anti-inflammatory, hence liquorice is used in most cough medicine and laxative-type medication. This tea also assists with weight loss.

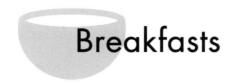

Breakfasts

Fruit salads

For good digestion and to avoid bloating and reflux, it is always best to group the following fruits together when making a fruit salad:

Citrus fruit salad
pineapple
oranges
mandarins
grapefruit

Stone fruit salad
mangoes
peaches
nectarines

Cut all the fruit into cubes and mix in a large bowl. Sprinkle with a little raw sugar or a drizzle of honey.

If you have a strong digestive system you can mix together any fruits you love, and then add the pulp of 2 passionfruit or a sprinkle of raw sugar and the juice of 1 orange.

Buckwheat pancakes makes approximately 16 pancakes

Buckwheat is a gluten-free 'energy' grain containing high amounts of a bioflavonoid called rutin, which helps strengthen blood vessels, especially with varicose veins and broken capillaries. Buckwheat is high in vitamins B_1 and B_6, niacin, folic acid and potassium. These pancakes make a great nutritious breakfast for the entire family, with your favourite fresh fruit or protein on top.

1 cup buckwheat flour
1 cup water (you can use milk instead of water for a thicker consistency)
1 tablespoon ground arrowroot
1 tablespoon light vegetable oil
¼ cup light olive oil for frying

In a bowl combine the flour, water, arrowroot and vegetable oil. Whisk the mixture until it is smooth and free of lumps.

Place a small frying pan over high heat and then add a little olive oil. Using a small ladle, pour in a small amount of the pancake mixture, approximately 1 tablespoon. Cook for 30 seconds or until small bubbles form in the mixture, then flip the pancake over and repeat on the second side until the pancake is brown all over. Drain the pancake on paper towel to remove any excess oil. Add more oil to the pan when necessary and cook until all the batter is used.

Wholemeal pancakes makes 10 pancakes

This is a perfect lunch dish served with a mixed green salad or Caesar salad (see page 148), or try the delicious fillings listed.

1 cup wholemeal or light white plain flour
1 free-range egg
1 cup skim milk
pinch of sea salt
¼ cup soda water
¼ cup olive oil, for frying

In the bowl of an electric mixer combine the flour, egg, milk and salt. Mix well until the mixture is very smooth; it should be slightly thick but a little runny. Transfer the mixture to a bowl and refrigerate for at least 1 hour.

Remove the mixture from the refrigerator and add the soda water. Stir gently as it froths a little.

Place a small frying pan over high heat and then add a little oil. Using a small ladle, pour in a small amount of the pancake mixture. Cook for 30 seconds or until small bubbles form in the mixture, then flip the pancake over and repeat on the second side until the pancake is brown all over. Drain the pancake on paper towel to remove any excess oil.

Try the following suggested fillings (these are especially good if you want to serve the pancakes at a party).

- Chopped smoked salmon or trout with dill and finely chopped cucumber
- Mushrooms sautéed with onions and garlic, with 1 teaspoon of light sour cream and seasoned with salt and pepper
- Finely chopped ham blended with pickled cucumber (you can add a little low-fat mayonnaise to help bind the mix)
- Finely chopped smoked salmon, dill and crème fraîche, with a little light sour cream and salmon roe on top of the rolled pancake

Oat porridge (the old-fashioned way) serves 3–4

Oats are the number-one grain for the nervous system and for restoring energy when you are run-down and stressed. They also lower cholesterol, strengthen heart muscles and raise the body temperature (ideal in cold weather). Eat oats daily for energy in high-stress situations such as sport and work.

Oats are very high in silicon (a mineral that helps bones and connective tissue) and phosphorus (a mineral that aids concentration; ideal for children), and they are also a great anti-ageing grain.

Start this recipe the night before for a truly authentic version.

1 cup whole organic rolled oats
5 cups water
½ teaspoon sea salt

In a saucepan combine the oats, water and salt. Soak overnight if you have the time. Bring to the boil and then reduce heat and simmer for 1–2 hours. The longer the oats simmer, the more delicious they become. Alternatively, you can cook the oats overnight in a rice cooker.

Serve with fruit, milk, raisins or prunes.

Oatmeal porridge (the faster way)   serves 3–4

1 cup organic rolled oats
2½–3 cups cold water

In a saucepan combine the oats and water. Cook, stirring, over a low heat for
5–8 minutes or until the mixture has thickened.

Homemade muesli   serves 4–5

*Muesli is filled with natural fibre and vitamins B and E. Lecithin contains choline and
inositol, which lower fats and cholesterol. Inositol is also vital in nerve functions.*

½ cup wheatgerm
½ cup whole organic rolled oats
¼ cup lecithin
½ cup sultanas
¼ cup raisins
½ cup slivered almonds
¼ teaspoon ground cinnamon (optional)
½ cup finely chopped dried apples or apricots (optional)

In a bowl combine all the ingredients. Mix well, then serve with yoghurt, milk, rice or soy
milk. Add cinnamon or dried fruit for extra flavour, if desired.
   Store leftovers in an airtight container in the refrigerator.

Energy porridge – a travelling breakfast   serves 1

Prepare this at night and store in a thermos until morning. I used this recipe every day when I was studying (I always enjoyed it with goat's milk and honey), so I highly recommend it for students, and for sportspeople.

1 tablespoon cracked organic wheat
2 teaspoons buckwheat
2 teaspoons organic rolled oats
boiling water

In a thermos combine the wheat, buckwheat and oats. Pour boiling water over the grains to cover by at least 3 cm and fasten the lid.

In the morning, serve the porridge with honey and milk. Making it in a thermos means you can take it to the office, or to the gym to eat after your early-morning exercise.

Scrambled curried eggs   serves 2

This is a nutritious, exotic way to serve eggs. Eggs are a complete protein and high in lecithin and choline. The yolk contains some cholesterol, but two eggs every second day for those who have normal cholesterol levels is suitable.

1 tablespoon vegetable oil
1 onion, finely chopped
1 handful fresh curry leaves, torn
1 green chilli, finely chopped
4 free-range eggs, beaten

Heat the oil in a frying pan, add the onion and cook until it is brown. Add the curry leaves, chilli and the beaten eggs and cook, stirring, for 1 minute or until the eggs are soft and light.

Remove curry leaves and serve eggs with toast or fresh yoghurt.

The healthy omelette   serves 1

This is a great way to serve eggs as a light meal.

Omelette

2 free-range eggs (if you have high cholesterol,
    use only the egg whites)
1 tablespoon water or low-fat milk
olive oil

Meat filling

1–2 slices of your favourite cooked cold
    meats, such as turkey, chicken or lamb,
    finely chopped

Cheese filling

1 tablespoon low-fat cottage cheese or 2–3 thin
slices mozzarella

Vegetarian filling 1

1 tomato, finely chopped
1 onion, finely chopped
4 fresh basil leaves

Vegetarian filling 2

1 medium mushroom, finely sliced
1 small carrot, finely chopped
1 small stick celery, finely sliced
1 leaf English spinach, washed and finely chopped

In a bowl whisk the eggs with the water or milk.

Add a little oil to a frying pan over medium heat. Pour in the egg mixture, reduce
heat to low and cook the omelette until the edge is curling a little; use a spatula to gently
lift the edge of the omelette and check that it is slightly brown underneath. Add your
favourite filling to one half of the omelette, then flip the other half over the top. Cook for
1 minute or until heated through, and serve.

Salads and dressings

Carrot and sultana salad   serves 2

Children love this because it is sweet, and it encourages them to eat carrots, which are high in antioxidants and enzymes. You can add some honey to this salad for children who have a sweet tooth. Children also love this with boiled eggs (a protein that contains lecithin, an important vitamin that assists certain brain pathways and development).

3 carrots, grated
juice of 1 orange
1 cup dried currants or sultanas
2 tablespoons desiccated coconut (optional)

In a salad bowl combine all the ingredients. Toss well and serve.

Rice salad   serves 4

This is a great salad to serve for lunch with a protein such as tuna, chicken or beans on the side or tossed through at the last minute. You can prepare this to take to work, with the protein in a separate container.

3 cups cooked brown rice, cooled (see page 178)

1 cup cooked peas

¼ cup deseeded and finely chopped red or green capsicum

2 tablespoons finely chopped fresh parsley

1 tablespoon toasted sesame seeds

2 tablespoons currants

2 tablespoons finely chopped chives (or green onions)

¼ cup Healthy French dressing (see page 153)

½ teaspoon ground turmeric

1 teaspoon ground cumin (optional)

In a large salad bowl combine the rice, peas, capsicum, parsley, sesame seeds, currants and chives. Drizzle the dressing over the salad and then sprinkle with the turmeric and cumin (if using) to serve.

My favourite Niçoise salad   serves 2

This is a very nutritious salad to throw together when you are tired and tempted to have takeaway. Vary the ingredients as you like, but remember that the principle stays the same: use one, two or three proteins with a base of lettuce and one or two steamed vegetables. The protein can be eggs, chicken or legumes such as chickpeas, lima beans or a can of mixed beans. A mix of two or three proteins gives added energy. You can change the potato to any steamed vegetable.

1 teaspoon balsamic vinegar
3 teaspoons extra-virgin olive oil
2 free-range eggs
4 baby new potatoes
½ lettuce, washed and chopped
1 × 100 g can tuna or salmon, drained
vegetable salt and freshly cracked black pepper, to taste

In a small jug combine the balsamic vinegar and oil.

Boil the eggs for 4 minutes, then remove them from the water and shell them. Set them aside to cool and then cut them in half.

Boil or steam the potatoes until just tender. (Use a sharp skewer to check.)

In a large bowl combine the egg, potato, lettuce and tuna/salmon. Mix these ingredients and then drizzle the dressing over the top. Season with vegetable salt and pepper and serve.

Jamie's lentil and bacon salad   serves 4

This recipe from my nephew Jamie Sach, a highly regarded sommelier in Adelaide, is a great accompaniment to barbecued meat, steamed fish and grilled chicken. Vegetarians can easily adapt this dish by leaving out the bacon and using vegetable stock.

3 cups brown lentils or green Puy-style lentils, soaked for several hours (overnight is ideal)

3 cups stock (see pages 159–160 for Vegetable stock and Chicken stock)

2 rashers bacon, fat trimmed, finely chopped

sea salt and freshly cracked black pepper, to taste

1 medium onion, finely chopped

2 sticks celery, finely chopped

1 large carrot, finely chopped

1 small bunch fresh parsley, roughly chopped

2 cloves garlic, crushed or finely chopped

2 tablespoons red-wine vinegar (balsamic will do but it is quite strong, so go easy)

2 tablespoons extra-virgin olive oil

Drain the lentils and transfer them to a saucepan with the stock and bacon. Bring to the boil, reduce heat to low and simmer, stirring occasionally, for 15–20 minutes or until the lentils only just begin to soften; the lentils cook by absorption and soak up the flavour of the stock, leaving only a little residual moisture (top with a little water if the mixture begins to dry). Season the lentils with salt and pepper and then put aside to cool.

Toss the onion, celery and carrot through the lentils and then mix through the parsley. In a jug combine the garlic, red-wine vinegar and olive oil and mix through the salad. Check seasoning and serve.

Avocado, mint and pea salad Serves 4–6

This salad is ideal for promoting healthy skin, as well as to combat arthritis (apple cider vinegar is excellent for joints) and a sluggish liver and bowel. The fresh mint assists digestion. You can use 1 drained 200 g can of green beans instead of fresh peas. Serve the salad with a protein or a vegetarian dish, such as steamed tofu on the side or grated cheese on top of the salad.

200 g freshly shelled peas
3 avocados, peeled and cut into cubes
½ cup chopped fresh mint leaves
2 tablespoons apple cider vinegar
1 tablespoon honey
1 chilli, finely chopped (optional)
1 small onion, finely sliced

Place the peas in a saucepan and cover them with water. Place them over heat and simmer for 15 minutes or until tender. Drain the peas and transfer them to a large salad bowl. Add the remaining ingredients and toss well.

Mixed salad with nuts   serves 4

Rocket contains chlorophyll, which aids absorption of iron in the blood. Walnuts are high in omega-6 fatty acids and excellent for lungs and poor circulation; they are delicious roasted. You can use pine nuts instead if you prefer. Tahini is made from sesame seeds, which are high in minerals and protein. If you don't like tahini, you can substitute the dressing by mixing 2 tablespoons olive oil and the juice of 1 lemon.

olive oil
1 cup walnuts, chopped, or ¼ cup pine nuts
1 small bunch mixed rocket and other salad leaves, washed and roughly chopped
1 small bunch watercress, leaves picked, washed and roughly chopped
2 tomatoes, cut into chunks
1 cucumber, cut into 1 cm slices
1–2 tablespoons tahini (see page 164)

Heat a little olive oil in a frying pan and sauté the nuts for 5 minutes or until brown. Remove from heat and place on a paper towel, to drain the oil.

In a salad bowl, combine the nuts, salad leaves, watercress, tomato and cucumber, then drizzle the tahini over the salad to serve.

Egg and asparagus salad   serves 2

This salad is quick, easy and nutritious for lunch or a light dinner. Eggs are a wonderful complete light protein. I often prepare this in the evening for lunch the following day. Add some boiled new potatoes for a carbohydrate, or eat with bread. You can also add other vegetables, such as steamed carrots or zucchini.

2 free-range eggs
½ bunch asparagus, washed and trimmed
2 tablespoons extra-virgin olive oil
½ teaspoon sea salt
1 medium avocado, peeled and cut into cubes
½ bunch rocket, washed and torn
¼ onion, finely chopped

Boil the eggs for 4 minutes, then drain and run under cold water for 2 minutes. Shell and cut into quarters.

Bring a saucepan of salted water to the boil. Add the asparagus and cook for 3–5 minutes or until tender. Drain the asparagus, cut into 2-cm lengths and then place in a bowl, adding the oil and salt.

In a large salad bowl combine the remaining ingredients. Add the egg and asparagus and toss thoroughly to serve.

Jamie's whole sardines with roasted garlic, olive and fennel salad   serves 2

Jamie, my much-loved nephew, created this wonderfully healthy dish. Sardines are very high in omega–3 oils, essential for lowering cholesterol and for dry skin irritations and cell membrane integrity in the brain. Fennel is a natural calmative, assisting digestion.

1 head garlic

olive oil, for baking

2 cups breadcrumbs

2 tablespoons finely chopped parsley

sea salt and freshly cracked black pepper

8–10 whole sardines, cleaned, rinsed
    and patted dry

1 bulb fennel, finely sliced

1 medium red onion, finely sliced

½ cup pitted black olives

1 tablespoon capers

1 tablespoon verjuice (or lemon juice
    or red-wine vinegar)

1 bunch flat-leaf parsley

2 tablespoons olive oil

1 lemon, cut into wedges

Preheat oven to 180°C.

Break up the head of garlic and roast the cloves whole with the skin on in a baking dish with a drizzle of olive oil for 15–20 minutes or until they soften. Remove the garlic from the oven (and increase oven temperature to 200°C) and set aside while you continue with the following steps.

Place the breadcrumbs in a large bowl and add the finely chopped parsley and a generous amount of salt and pepper. Stuff the cavity of the sardines with some of the breadcrumb mixture, then roll them in it to coat thoroughly.

Line the sardines in a lightly oiled baking dish and bake for 10–12 minutes (alternatively you can shallow-fry the sardines in olive oil for a crunchier texture).

Meanwhile, combine the fennel and red onion in a large bowl. Add the olives, capers, roasted garlic cloves, verjuice, some whole parsley leaves and 2 tablespoons olive oil, and season with salt and pepper. Arrange the salad on a serving plate and place the whole cooked sardines on top. Serve with wedges of lemon.

Couscous salad   serves 4

With its herbs and flowers, this light grain salad looks great in summer on the table with barbecued seafood. It is filling, but not as heavy as brown rice. Couscous is high in vitamins, minerals and fibre, especially vitamins B_1, B_2 and B_6, niacin, magnesium and manganese, phosphorus and potassium. It aids in stabilising blood sugar and energy levels and is useful for hypoglycaemia and hormone-related mood swings, as well as providing energy for athletes and children, especially children who are overweight. If edible flowers are unavailable, add some sprigs of fresh herbs instead.

2 cups couscous

3 cups hot water

1 tablespoon lemon juice

juice of 1 lemon

1 small bunch edible flowers, such as zucchini flowers or nasturtiums, washed (optional)

100 g roasted pine nuts, almonds or cashews, chopped

1 tablespoon chopped fresh coriander or parsley

¼ cup chopped fresh mint

1 cup dried apricots, sliced

2 tablespoons finely grated lemon zest

In a large bowl combine the couscous, hot water and the tablespoon of lemon juice. Stir and set aside, covered, to soak for 10–15 minutes.

Meanwhile, place the lemon juice in a medium stainless-steel mixing bowl – it should be large enough to just hold all the couscous. Press some of the edible flowers (if using) onto the base of the bowl.

When the couscous has soaked up the water, add the nuts, coriander or parsley, mint, apricot and lemon zest, and mix well with a fork, fluffing the couscous as you stir. Transfer the couscous to the bowl containing the lemon juice and the flowers, and press the mixture down flat, flush with the top of the bowl. Firmly hold a flat plate over the top of the bowl and invert it to turn out the couscous salad with the flowers. If this sounds a little ambitious, simply serve the salad straight from the bowl – it won't look as pretty, but it will taste just as good.

Decorate the salad with the remaining flowers and refrigerate until ready to serve.

My favourite Caesar salad   serves 4

This salad should be served with a simple protein such as grilled fish, chicken or meat, or a legume dish. Both tasty and gentle on the digestion, this salad is a hit for entertaining at home.

1 iceberg lettuce, outer leaves removed and
    lettuce washed and drained in a colander
3 hardboiled free-range eggs, quartered
4 slices prosciutto
½ teaspoon chopped fresh oregano
olive oil, for frying
2 tablespoons shaved parmesan
freshly cracked black pepper
1 handful chopped fresh parsley

Croutons (or use ½ packet ready-made croutons)
2 cloves garlic, finely chopped
½ teaspoon paprika
½ cup olive oil
6 slices bread, cut into cubes (crusts removed)

Dressing
¼ cup balsamic vinegar or white-wine vinegar
½ cup extra-virgin olive oil
1 teaspoon Dijon mustard
juice of ½ lemon
3–4 anchovy fillets
sea salt and freshly cracked black pepper, to taste

To make the croutons, heat the oil in a frying pan for 30 seconds and then add the garlic and paprika. Add the bread cubes and mix until the cubes are well coated. Transfer to a microwave-proof dish. Microwave for 3–5 minutes (or you can bake them on an oven tray at 180°C for 15 minutes) until the cubes are lightly browned. Set aside.

In a blender mix the vinegar, olive oil, mustard, lemon juice and anchovies until the mixture is thick but runny. Season with salt and pepper to taste and set the dressing aside while you prepare the salad.

Tear the lettuce leaves into pieces and place in a salad bowl. Add the eggs to the bowl.

Add a little oil to a frying pan and place over medium heat. Add the prosciutto slices and then sprinkle with the oregano. Cook for 5 minutes or until crispy, then remove the prosciutto and allow it to cool a little. When it has cooled, break it into chunky pieces and then add to the salad bowl.

Pour the dressing over the salad and then scatter the parmesan over the top. Sprinkle with black pepper, parsley and croutons and toss gently before serving.

Butter bean, potato and spinach salad   serves 4

This salad is a perfect combination of protein (beans), carbohydrate (potato) and a green vegetable, with a healthy dressing. This can be a complete meal in summer or served as a side salad to a fish or chicken dish. It's great for those who are cutting back on meat and chicken and want to increase energy while keeping weight down.

Salad

4 medium potatoes, peeled and quartered

4 salad onions, halved lengthways

freshly cracked black pepper, to taste

1 × 400 g can butter beans, drained

100 g baby spinach leaves, washed

2 cloves garlic, crushed

Dressing

2 tablespoons balsamic vinegar

1 tablespoon wholegrain mustard (optional)

1 tablespoon honey

2 tablespoons chopped fresh parsley

Preheat oven to 180°C.

Arrange the potato and onion on a baking tray. Sprinkle with pepper (don't use any oils) and bake until the potatoes are soft and slightly brown – about 1 hour.

While the potatoes and salad onions are baking, combine the dressing ingredients in a bowl. Mix well, then set the dressing aside.

Transfer the hot potato and salad onion to a salad bowl and add the remaining ingredients. Mix well, drizzle the dressing over and serve immediately.

Chickpea and avocado salad   serves 4

Chickpeas are a nutritious legume, and are higher in protein than eggs and many meats. They are also high in B group vitamins, calcium, iron, zinc and potassium. Avocado is rich in omega-6 fatty acids for healthy skin and hair.

Salad

1 medium carrot, finely sliced

2 medium zucchini, finely sliced

2 cups cooked or drained canned chickpeas
    (about 2 × 400 g cans)

1 onion, finely chopped

½ cup black olives, pitted and chopped

2 avocados, peeled and sliced

Dressing

2 tablespoons tamari

1 clove garlic, chopped

1 tablespoon honey

juice of ½ lemon

1 tablespoon roasted slivered almonds, sesame
seeds or pine nuts (optional)

In a jug combine the dressing ingredients. Mix well.

Boil or steam the carrot and zucchini slices, along with the chickpeas, for 5 minutes, then drain and transfer them to a salad bowl.

Add the remaining salad ingredients and toss gently. Drizzle the dressing over and toss before serving.

Beetroot and asparagus salad   serves 4

Beetroot helps cleanse the spleen, liver and pancreas. Asparagus contains asparagine, which helps the kidneys eliminate excess water. It is also high in vitamin A (for those with lung problems) and potassium (for arthritis sufferers).

Beetroot and asparagus are used widely in cancer clinics for their nutritional properties and healing effects in cleansing free radicals from the body. This salad is excellent for those with joint, liver, lung or spleen problems.

1 bunch (approximately 400 g) fresh beetroot, washed
2 bunches asparagus, washed and trimmed
1 tablespoon balsamic vinegar or lemon juice
1 red capsicum, deseeded and thinly sliced
1 tablespoon chopped fresh chives
1 tablespoon sesame seeds, toasted

Steam or boil the beetroot for 1 hour or until tender (cooking time will depend on the size of the beetroot). Remove from water and use a knife to help you peel off the skin, which will have become loose. Set the beetroot aside to cool slightly, then cut it into slices or cubes and transfer them to a salad bowl.

Steam or boil the asparagus for 5 minutes, then rinse under cold water. Transfer to the salad bowl with the beetroot and combine.

Drizzle the balsamic vinegar or lemon juice over the beetroot and asparagus, and mix in the capsicum. Sprinkle the chives and sesame seeds over the top and serve.

SALAD DRESSINGS

You can make any salad even more delicious if you choose fresh, healthy ingredients to include in the dressing. Try apple cider vinegar, fresh lemon juice and lime juice mixed with any cold-pressed oil you love.

Paw paw dressing   makes 1 cup

2 cups peeled, seeded and chopped paw paw
2 tablespoons lemon juice

Blend all the ingredients in an electric mixer and serve immediately.

Healthy French dressing   makes about 2 cups

1 cup extra-virgin olive oil
¼ cup freshly squeezed lemon juice
½ cup apple cider vinegar
1 clove garlic, crushed (optional)
2 teaspoons honey
freshly cracked black pepper, to taste (optional)

With an electric mixer, blend all the ingredients. Store the dressing in an airtight container in the refrigerator for up to 2 days.

French tomato dressing   makes 1 cup

1 cup tomato juice (or Simple tomato sauce, see page 175)

1 tablespoon lemon juice

2 tablespoons chopped fresh basil

With an electric mixer, blend all the ingredients. Store the dressing in an airtight container in the refrigerator for up to 2 days.

Soups and stocks

Barley soup   serves 4

Barley helps increase energy and supplies nourishment for active people who need a carbohydrate and vegetable boost.

1 tablespoon olive oil
¼ onion, chopped
4 carrots, grated
2 parsnips, peeled and chopped
2 litres water
1 cup pearl barley
⅓ teaspoon grated ginger (optional)
sea salt, to taste
½ bunch fresh parsley, chopped

Heat the oil in a saucepan over medium heat. Add the onion, carrot and parsnip, and sauté for 5 minutes or until tender. Add the water, barley and ginger, then reduce heat and simmer for 1½ hours, stirring occasionally. Season with salt and add the parsley to serve.

Cauliflower and broccoli soup   serves 6

My friend Suzie serves this soup at some of her wonderful parties. Cauliflower and broccoli contain antioxidants. This hearty soup is ideal for an entrée for dinner parties as well as served in winter with chunks of hot wholemeal bread.

2 tablespoons butter

1 large head of cauliflower, finely chopped

1 large head of broccoli, finely chopped

1 bunch spring onions, chopped

1 teaspoon rock salt and 1 large pinch ground white pepper

2 pinches cayenne pepper (optional)

2 litres Vegetable or Chicken stock (see pages 159–160)

2 free-range egg yolks

¼ cup light cream

4 sprigs fresh parsley and ½ bunch fresh chives, finely chopped and combined

½ cup yoghurt, to serve

In a large saucepan, melt the butter over medium heat. Add the cauliflower, broccoli and spring onion and stir for 5–8 minutes or until soft. Season with salt, pepper and cayenne pepper if using. Add the stock and simmer for 40 minutes. Allow the soup to cool a little, then transfer to a blender. Purée, then transfer back to the saucepan and reheat.

As the soup is heating, beat the egg yolks with the cream in a bowl. Add this mixture to the hot soup very slowly, whisking constantly to ensure the eggs do not become scrambled. Garnish with the parsley–chive mixture and yoghurt, and serve.

Minestrone soup   serves 6

This nutritious soup may be portioned and frozen so you can eat it anytime or use as a snack when you arrive home late. It's great with crusty bread.

1 kg chuck steak and/or ½ free-range chicken

1 teaspoon sea salt

2 medium onions, chopped

3 cloves garlic, chopped

3 medium potatoes, peeled and chopped

3 large carrots, chopped

4 sticks celery, chopped

1 handful peas

1 handful green beans, chopped

3 large tomatoes, chopped

1 × 200 g can bean mix, drained

1 bunch English spinach, washed and chopped (optional)

200 g lentils

½ head broccoli or cauliflower, chopped

4 slices bread

2 tablespoons grated parmesan

sea salt, extra, and freshly cracked black pepper, to taste

Fill a large saucepan with 4–5 litres of water and add the chuck steak and chicken. Bring to the boil and boil for at least 2 hours to create your own broth.

Add the salt, then reduce heat to a simmer and transfer the chuck steak and chicken to a chopping board, leaving the saucepan on the stove. Remove the skin from the chicken. Cut the chuck steak and chicken into cubes and return them to the saucepan. Add the onion, garlic, potato, carrot, celery, peas, beans, tomato, bean mix, spinach, lentils, broccoli or cauliflower. Simmer for 2 hours.

When the soup is ready, toast the bread and then cut it into cubes. Sprinkle the cheese over the bread and grill for 1–2 minutes or until the cheese browns.

Season the soup with salt and pepper and serve with the cheesy croutons.

Cleansing noodle soup   serves 2

This is excellent during a detox; alternate this with the Minestrone soup on page 157.

1 litre Vegetable stock (see opposite)
1 carrot, chopped
1 spring onion, chopped
2 cups dried noodles (of your choice)
1 small bunch bok choy or ½ bunch spinach (or a mix of both), washed and chopped

In a large saucepan combine the stock, carrot and onion. Place over a high heat and bring to a boil. Add the noodles, reduce heat to low, and simmer until the noodles are cooked. Add the greens and cook until they are tender then serve.

VEGETABLE, FISH AND CHICKEN STOCKS

Homemade stocks are nutritious and far superior to commercial stocks. Use however much you need for a recipe at the time and then freeze the rest in containers.

Vegetable stock   makes about 3 litres

Kombu (seaweed), found in your health food store, is part of the kelp family and is great in soups, casseroles, salads and sautés. It assists digestion.

2 medium onions, quartered
2 large carrots, chopped
4–5 sticks celery, chopped
1 leek, washed and chopped
6 cm piece kombu (for extra flavour)
4 litres water

In a large saucepan combine all the ingredients and place over low heat. Simmer for 45 minutes. Strain, remove the kombu (it can be re-used) and throw the vegetables on the compost heap. Freeze the stock in airtight containers for future use.

Fish stock   makes about 3 litres

2 large fish heads or 1 kg prawn shells and heads
1 bunch fresh parsley, roughly chopped
2 large onions, chopped
3 cloves garlic, chopped
2 tablespoons fish sauce
6 cm piece kombu (optional)
4 litres water

In a large saucepan combine all the ingredients and bring to the boil, then reduce heat and simmer for 30–40 minutes. Strain the stock and discard all the solids (you may need to use a fine sieve). Skim any fat from the surface. Freeze the stock in airtight containers for future use.

Chicken stock   makes about 3 litres

1 medium-size free-range chicken, washed
2 medium onions, roughly chopped
2 large carrots, chopped
1 medium leek, washed and chopped
3–4 sticks celery, chopped
4 litres water

In a large saucepan combine all the ingredients and bring to the boil, then reduce heat and simmer for 1½–2 hours. Strain the stock and cool in the refrigerator. Remove any fat from the surface. Freeze the stock in airtight containers for future use. Use the chicken in sandwiches, soups or a risotto.

Snacks, sandwiches and side dishes

Healthy snacks for twenty-first-century living have become rare. Unfortunately, sugar-loaded 'health' bars have replaced simple, quick and nutritious home-cooked snacks.

People with low blood sugar levels (hypoglycaemia) need healthy snacks every 3–4 hours. Growing active children, sportspeople, students and those who work in high-pressure industries requiring 'brain energy' also need to snack.

Try the recipes in this section or some of the following quick options.

Savoury snacks

- A handful of almonds, cashews or macadamias with a handful of raisins
- Vita-Weat or Ryvita biscuits with a slice of chicken, ham, beef (plus a touch of wholegrain mustard) and a slice of tomato with black pepper, or a small can of tuna or salmon
- A bowl of vegetable soup
- A toasted sandwich on wholemeal grainy bread
- 1–2 boiled eggs
- A sushi roll and miso soup

Sweet snacks

- 2 pieces of fresh fruit
- Yoghurt with honey or fruit
- A slice of wholemeal bread topped with tahini (see page 164) and honey
- A wholemeal muffin
- A slice of wholemeal cake
- Poached fruit and yoghurt
- A fruit, milk and yoghurt smoothie (you can add 1 tablespoon whey powder for extra energy)
- A good-quality muesli bar (your health store can make a recommendation)

If you are watching your waistline, stay with protein snacks and fresh fruits, not cakes, biscuits or sweets.

Chickpea spread   makes about 2 cups

Chickpeas are a superb complete protein and are at their best as a spread or used in soups and casseroles. Children love chickpeas when they are made into a dip with garlic and onions, which have an antibacterial effect against colds and flus in winter. This spread is wonderful served on whole wheat bread, Lebanese bread or Vegetable rissoles (see page 198), or as a dip with raw vegetables. You need to soak dried chickpeas overnight.

2 cups dried chickpeas, soaked overnight in water (or you can use 2 × 400 g cans chickpeas)

½ cup lemon juice

1 tablespoon ground cumin or coriander

2 cloves garlic, crushed

1 medium onion, chopped

¼ cup water or apple juice

1–2 tablespoons tahini (optional; see page 164)

Rinse the chickpeas and, if using dried chickpeas, simmer until soft (about 1–2 hours). Combine all the ingredients in an electric blender. Blend until you have a smooth paste, then cover and store in the refrigerator for up to 2 weeks.

Tahini (sesame seed butter)   makes about ½ cup

Sesame seeds are high in calcium, phosphorus and potassium, which is great for vegetarians. This versatile butter is great as a spread on wholemeal crackers, and is delicious used in dips.

You can soak sesame seeds overnight and lightly pan-roast them before grinding if you need to sprinkle them over salad. Sesame seed oil is delicious for flavouring any dish or used to sauté vegetables.

1 cup sesame seeds
2 teaspoons linseed oil

Combine the sesame seeds and oil in the bowl of a food processor. Blend the ingredients into a paste, then cover and place in the refrigerator. This will keep, covered in the refrigerator, for up to 10 days.

Avocado dip   makes about 2 cups

Avocado contains omega-6 fatty acids, which are excellent for dry skin. Children enjoy this served with wholemeal bread, water biscuits or slices of raw carrot, celery and cucumber as an alternative to sweets after school.

2 large ripe avocados, peeled and chopped
2 tomatoes, finely chopped
¼ teaspoon vegetable salt
2 tablespoons lemon or lime juice
1 clove garlic, crushed (optional)
pinch of chilli (optional)

Place avocado in a bowl and mash with a fork until smooth. Add the remaining ingredients and mix well.

Jacket potato   serves 1

The potato is a wonderful form of carbohydrate. Just beneath its skin is a rich variety of minerals (especially potassium, magnesium and phosphorus), so eating a potato in its jacket with fillings on top is a balanced and healthy snack. Alternatively, you can add this vegetable to any dish. Teenagers and children love jacket potatoes, and they are far superior to French fries.

1 potato per person
dob of butter, to serve
sea salt, to serve

Preheat oven to 180°C.

Wash the skin of the potato and then place the potato on a lined baking tray. Bake for 45 minutes or until the potato is soft in the centre (pierce with a skewer to test). Alternatively, cook the potato in a microwave for approximately 5 minutes. (The time will depend on the size of the potato.)

Transfer the potato to a serving plate. Slice the potato open or cut the top off and add a dob of butter and a sprinkle of salt, followed by your favourite topping. Try the following suggestions; you can scoop out the hot potato flesh, combine it with one of these mixtures, pile it back into its jacket and briefly return to the oven to warm through.

- Finely chopped onion mixed with a small can of tuna or salmon, a little extra-virgin olive oil and sea salt.
- Finely chopped tomato mixed with a touch of chilli or a finely chopped clove of garlic.
- Creamed cheese and chopped chives.
- Grated tasty cheese, melted under the grill (perfect for hungry teenagers).
- Snipped fresh chives and a dob of sour cream.

Tasty sandwiches with lavash or Lebanese bread

These sandwiches are low in carbohydrates and are excellent for those on a yeast-free diet, as well as anyone trying to lose weight, or who suffers from bloating. These sandwiches also appeal to children who are bored with standard sandwiches, especially if you slice them into 4–6 cm rolls.

Suggested fillings

Meat

chicken or ham slices

wholegrain or Dijon mustard, or low-fat
    mayonnaise

lettuce or rocket

Vegetarian

hummus

grated carrot

lettuce

Lentils

cold cooked red lentils

grated carrot

chopped capsicum

Tuna

well-drained tuna

sliced onion

grated carrot

Arrange your chosen fillings on one side of a piece of lavash or Lebanese bread and roll, then cut into 4–6 cm strips. Do not use fillings that go soggy – such as beetroot and tomato – if you are filling a lunchbox with sandwiches that will be eaten in several hours' time.

Cheese, tomato and basil pizza   makes 4 small pizzas

A fresh homemade pizza is a great option on a weekend. Well-ripened tomatoes, although acidic, will alkalise the blood, helping ease rheumatism. Large amounts of tomato upset calcium metabolism, so use sparingly if you suffer from arthritis or kidney stones.

Pizza base

2 cups pizza flour

1 cup warm water

1 cube fresh yeast (you will find this in your
    health food store)

2 tablespoons olive oil

pinch of sea salt

Topping

1 × 400 g can chopped peeled tomatoes

1 clove garlic, crushed

1 teaspoon dried oregano

½ bunch fresh basil

pinch sea salt

mozzarella or parmesan, grated

To make the pizza base, place the flour in a large bowl and make a well in the centre. In a jug combine the water and yeast, stirring until the yeast has dissolved. Pour into the flour well, then add the oil and salt and mix with a wooden spoon until a dough forms.

Wash and dry your hands, then lightly flour your benchtop. Place the dough on the bench and knead: use the heel of your hand to push it gently away, then pull it back – it should take 5–10 minutes for the dough to become smooth and elastic. Return to the bowl, cover with a clean tea towel and set aside in a warm place for 1–1½ hours or until it has doubled in size.

While the dough is rising, combine the tomatoes, garlic, oregano, basil and salt in a bowl. Preheat oven to 200°C and grease 2 oven trays.

Roll the dough into circles and place on the trays (2 pizzas per tray) and cover each with tomato mixture, followed by the mozzarella or parmesan. Bake for 20 minutes or until the cheese has melted and the bases are crisp.

My favourite antipasto platter   serves 4

This is wonderful for parties or as a starter for dinner; it is also very nourishing and attractive. Serve with freshly cut baguettes or bread rolls on the side.

12 slices salami
16 black olives
8 slices ham
8 sundried tomatoes
2 medium bocconcini, sliced
12 fresh basil leaves

Arrange the ingredients in rows on a large serving platter, decorated with the basil leaves.

Potato and sweet potato wedges   serves 2

This is a great carbohydrate snack to fill up on. Combined with a protein dip such as chickpea spread or avocado dip, it is an ideal snack for the family, especially children when they get home from school or even for a teenager's party. I do not recommend this dish for diabetics, however, because sweet potatoes are high in natural sugars.

2 large potatoes, washed and cut into long wedges (leave skins on)
1 large sweet potato, peeled and cut into wedges
2 tablespoons extra-virgin olive oil, for baking
sea salt and freshly cracked black pepper, to taste

Preheat oven to 180°C.

Line a baking tray with baking paper.

Dry the wedges with paper towel, then toss them in a large bowl with oil and season with salt and pepper and spread the wedges out on the baking tray. Bake for 1 hour or until the wedges are crisp on the outside.

Sprinkle some salt over the wedges and serve them with your favourite dip.

For something different, spread a little wholegrain mustard over the wedges, or coat them with mixed herbs such as dried oregano or paprika before cooking.

Potato, onion and cheese bake   serves 4

This dish is delicious served with grilled fish, fresh prawns or a simple grilled fillet steak – it's my favourite side dish in winter.

butter, for greasing casserole dish
5 large potatoes, peeled and finely sliced lengthways
3 onions, finely sliced
200 g tasty cheese, grated
sea salt and freshly cracked black pepper, to taste
1½ cups milk
1 tablespoon butter, for melting

Preheat oven to 180°C.

Grease a medium baking or casserole dish (a rectangular one works best) with a dob of butter. Cover the bottom of the dish with a layer of potato slices. Melt 1 tablespoon butter in a small saucepan over low heat, then using a brush spread a little butter evenly over the potato slices. Add a layer of onion slices and sprinkle some cheese and salt and pepper over the top. Repeat these rows until you have used all the ingredients, finishing with the cheese.

Add 2–3 dobs of butter to the top cheese layer and pour over the milk. Cover with foil and bake for 45 minutes, removing the foil in the last 10 minutes so the cheese browns. Serve immediately.

Couscous   serves 2

Couscous is a tiny grain made from wheat that is light and simple to prepare. High in niacin, fibre, calcium and magnesium, this grain can be used instead of pasta, brown rice or buckwheat as a base for serving with stir-fries.

1 cup couscous
2½ cups warm water
pinch of sea salt

Place all the ingredients in a saucepan and place over low heat. Simmer for 1 minute and then let it stand, covered, for 10 minutes or until most of the water has soaked into the grain. Use a fork to gently fluff the grains until they are soft before serving.

Buckwheat   serves 2–4

Buckwheat is a wonder energy grain with a delicious sweet and nutty flavour, but it is unfortunately highly overlooked in Western society. It is gluten-free and contains a bioflavonoid called rutin, which strengthens capillaries, blood vessels and is now claimed to be highly beneficial as an antidote to radiation. Buckwheat is an important grain for those with cardiovascular diseases, varicose veins, poor circulation, diabetes and intolerances to wheat and gluten. Try to eat some 2–3 times a week. You can also try Japanese soba noodles, which are made from buckwheat flour.

If you haven't tried buckwheat before, the tastiest option is kasha, a toasted reddish-brown buckwheat you can buy from health stores. Kasha is one of the few grains that are alkaline, making it good for those with arthritis, ulcers, itchy skin conditions and heartburn.

2½ cups water
1 cup toasted buckwheat (kasha)
½ onion, chopped (optional)
½ teaspoon sea salt

Pour the water into a large saucepan and bring to the boil. Add the buckwheat, onion (if you would like some extra flavour) and salt, reduce heat and simmer, covered, for 10–15 minutes or until the grain is soft. Drain any excess water and then transfer the mixture to serving bowls.

To add extra flavour, try a splash of soy sauce, a dob of butter or a tablespoon of olive oil mixed through the grains.

Tasty grated onion and potato cakes   serves 2

Not only are these cakes nutritious and tasty, children will love helping you make them. They are delicious served with fish or a meat dish.

2 potatoes, peeled and grated
2 zucchini, grated
2 carrots, grated
2 medium onions, grated
2 tablespoons extra-virgin olive oil

In a bowl combine all the vegetables and mix well. Add a little of the oil to a frying pan over medium heat. Form the mixture into small–medium flat potato cakes and sauté for 3–4 minutes on each side or until browned all over.

Simple tomato sauce   serves 6 (or 4 with some left over to freeze)

This simple sauce is wonderful with any pasta.

olive oil
1 medium onion, finely chopped
2 cloves garlic, chopped
3 × 400 g cans peeled crushed tomatoes, or 8 fresh large tomatoes, quartered
1 teaspoon brown or white sugar
½ bunch fresh basil, roughly chopped

Heat the oil in a frying pan and place over medium heat. Add the onion and garlic, and sauté until the onion is translucent and soft. Add the tomatoes and then refill one of the empty cans with water and add to the pan. Simmer for 2 minutes, then add the sugar and basil and simmer for 1 hour, stirring occasionally.

When serving you can add a little cream (1 teaspoon per person) or some finely chopped mushrooms for extra flavour.

Mashed potato   serves 4

I always tell my clients not to be afraid of mashed, steamed or boiled potatoes; the potato is a healthy carbohydrate and is very alkaline and soothing to upset stomachs, peptic ulcers and irritable bowels. Keep the skin on if possible to retain all the minerals. Mashed potatoes make the perfect carbohydrate alternative to bread, especially if you are allergic to wheat and grains.

4 medium–large potatoes, washed and halved
sea salt and freshly cracked black pepper, to taste
2 teaspoons unsalted butter
½ cup milk (optional)

Bring a large saucepan of water to the boil. Add the potatoes and boil for 10–15 minutes, or until the potatoes are soft. Drain the potatoes, reserving 1 tablespoon of the cooking water.

Transfer the potatoes to a large bowl. Add the reserved cooking water and the butter and milk (if using), and mash to a smooth consistency. Season with salt and pepper and serve. This is delicious with meat and fish.

Brown rice   serves 2

The outer shell of brown rice is high in B vitamins and therefore important in our busy lifestyles to balance stress, energy fluctuations, nervousness, depression and for natural fibre. It is excellent eaten daily for those with yeast and gluten intolerances. It must be chewed thoroughly and I always recommend a simple protein and vegetable dish on top. This recipe makes about 3 cups of cooked rice.

1 cup short-grain brown rice (organic is best)
3 cups cold water or Vegetable stock (see page 159)
½ teaspoon sea salt

Wash and drain the rice and place it in a saucepan with the water and salt. Cover the saucepan and bring to a rapid boil, then reduce the heat and simmer for 30–45 minutes with the lid on or until most of the liquid has been absorbed. Drain off any excess liquid.

Remove the lid, stir carefully and leave the mixture to rest, covered, for 5 minutes before serving.

Notes
- For Thai dishes, use jasmine rice.
- For Indian dishes, use basmati rice.
- For risotto, use arborio rice.

Sautéed potatoes   serves 3–4

These are wonderful served with chicken, lamb or steak.

12 new baby potatoes (leave skins on)
olive oil
2 cloves garlic, crushed
1 teaspoon fresh rosemary leaves
sea salt and freshly cracked black pepper, to taste

Bring a large saucepan of water to the boil. Add the potatoes and boil for 10 minutes or until just cooked, then remove and drain. Set potatoes aside to cool.

Add the oil and garlic to a frying pan over low heat and sauté for 1 minute. Add the cooled potatoes and rosemary, season with salt and pepper and sauté for 1 minute. Serve immediately.

Main meals

Pan-fried salmon serves 2

This simple dish is especially good for those with high cholesterol, who suffer from eczema or PMT, or need to lose weight. It is also wonderful for children's brain development. You can also use tuna or kingfish instead of salmon.

2 teaspoons rock salt
2 salmon fillets
olive oil
juice of 1 lemon

Spread the salt evenly over both sides of the salmon.

Place the oil and lemon juice in a frying pan and heat over medium heat. Add the salmon and cook on each side for 4 minutes or until cooked to your liking – most people prefer salmon a little pink in the middle.

Serve with three steamed vegetables, such as carrots, potato and broccoli, for an extra antioxidant boost.

Angela's spinach and cheese bake   serves 4

My sister Angela makes this dish for her 9- and 11-year-old boys. It provides protein and calcium, and it encourages children to eat spinach.

butter, for cooking
½ cup chopped broccoli
½ cup chopped cauliflower
1 tablespoon pumpkin seeds
1 tablespoon soy sauce
2 cloves garlic, chopped
1 bunch fresh spinach, washed and stems
    removed, and finely chopped

200 g tasty cheese, grated
4 potatoes, thinly sliced (leave skins on)
1 medium zucchini, thinly sliced
2 tomatoes, sliced
2 tablespoons tasty cheese, grated, extra
2 cups Vegetable stock (see page 159)
2 tablespoons sesame seeds

Preheat oven to 180°C.

Heat a little butter in a frying pan over medium heat. Add the broccoli, cauliflower, pumpkin seeds, soy sauce and garlic, and sauté until the vegetables are just brown.

While the vegetables are cooking, grease the bottom of a casserole dish (34 × 25 cm; 6 cm deep). In a bowl mix the spinach with the cheese, then transfer the mixture to the casserole dish. Top with a layer of potato slices. Layer the stir-fried vegetable mixture over the potato, then arrange the zucchini and tomato slices on top and add the extra cheese. Sprinkle the sesame seeds over the top, then pour in the vegetable stock.

Bake for 40–50 minutes. Serve with a salad.

Rustic country Italian pasta   serves 4

My Italian friend Maria serves this pasta dish to hungry teenagers or when feeding a big family gathering. It is tasty, healthy and easy to prepare.

10 g dried porcini mushrooms – about 1 sachet
400 g dried spaghetti
½ cup olive oil
2 cloves garlic, sliced
1 × 185 g can tuna in oil, drained
100 g pancetta, finely chopped (optional)
1 × 400 g can diced tomatoes

Add the porcini mushrooms to a cup of warm water and leave to soak for 20 minutes.

Bring a large saucepan of salted water to the boil. Add the spaghetti and boil for 6 minutes or until al dente.

While the spaghetti is cooking, heat the oil in a frying pan over high heat. Add the garlic, drained porcini, tuna, pancetta and tomatoes, and cook, stirring, for 5 minutes.

Drain the spaghetti and divide among serving bowls. Pour the sauce over the spaghetti and serve with a salad on the side.

Maria's peasant-style chicken with rosemary   serves 4

This is a country dish from my friend Maria. It makes a tasty meal for all the family, especially on a cold winter evening. Rosemary is an antioxidant herb for the brain. This rustic casserole is wonderful served with steamed green beans and crusty bread to mop up the juices.

4 free-range chicken marylands
3 cloves garlic, chopped
1 onion, sliced
½ bunch fresh parsley leaves, chopped
½ bunch fresh rosemary leaves, chopped
sea salt and freshly cracked black pepper, to taste
3 medium potatoes, washed and halved
3 tablespoons extra-virgin olive oil
375 ml dry white wine
3 tablespoons grated parmesan

Preheat oven to 180°C.

Place the chicken in a medium-sized baking dish.

In a bowl combine the garlic, onion, parsley and rosemary, then sprinkle the mixture over the chicken and season with salt and pepper.

Wedge the potato halves between the chicken pieces, then drizzle oil over the top. Pour the wine over and then sprinkle with parmesan. Cover with foil and bake for 1 hour.

Remove the foil then return the dish to the oven for 5 minutes to brown the parmesan.

Serve with steamed or boiled green beans and crusty bread.

Tuna macaroni   serves 4

This pasta dish is quick and easy to prepare for the family; it can also be a snack for hungry children and teenagers after school. Tuna is high in omega-6 fatty acids, and this dish is excellent for dry skin, arthritis and weak digestion. Parmesan adds flavour and is high in calcium.

400 g macaroni
1 × 375 g can tuna in oil, drained
1 tablespoon butter
2 tablespoons grated parmesan
sea salt and freshly cracked black pepper, to taste

Bring a large saucepan of salted water to the boil. Add the macaroni and boil for 5 minutes or until al dente.

While the pasta is cooking, combine the tuna, butter and parmesan in a bowl.

Drain the pasta and then return it to the saucepan. Add the tuna mixture and stir gently to combine. Season with salt and pepper and serve.

Spinach and rice   serves 4–6

This dish is wonderfully gentle for those with an upset stomach, heartburn or anaemia. Spinach is high in vitamin A and folic acid, and contains some calcium, magnesium and other trace minerals. Rice is gluten-free and helps to line the stomach. Children and teenagers also enjoy this dish and you can make it a complete meal by serving it with fish, chicken or legumes.

1½ tablespoons extra-virgin olive oil
½ bunch spring onions, chopped
1 bunch fresh dill, chopped
1 bunch coarse spinach, washed and shredded with coarse stems removed
3½ cups water
1 cup long-grain rice (white or brown)
sea salt and freshly cracked black pepper, to taste
juice of 1 lemon

Add the oil to a saucepan over a low heat. Add the spring onion and dill and sauté for 5 minutes. Add the spinach and 1 cup water and stir for 2 minutes. Add remaining water and the rice and season with salt and pepper. Increase heat to medium and cook for 15 minutes. Remove the saucepan from the heat and cover with a tight-fitting lid. Leave to steam in its juices for 5 minutes for white rice or 15–20 minutes for brown rice, then pour over the lemon juice and serve.

Chicken and vegetable casserole   serves 4

The whole family will love this dish – and so will the cook, as the oven does all the work. If you like, add some broccoli to the casserole 10 minutes before it is ready, or steam some green vegetables while the casserole is cooking. For variety you can add some chopped ginger, or 1–2 teaspoons chopped rosemary or some fresh basil leaves.

4 free-range chicken breasts

4 carrots, roughly chopped

2 large onions, cut into 6–8 wedges

3 cloves garlic, chopped

4 medium potatoes, washed and cut into quarters

4 tomatoes, cut into 4–6 wedges

½ cup olive oil

1½ cups water

1 teaspoon sea salt

½ teaspoon freshly cracked black pepper

1–2 tablespoons chopped fresh parsley

1 tablespoon chopped ginger (optional)

Preheat oven to 190°C.

Arrange the chicken, carrot, onion, garlic, potato and tomato in a large baking dish. Splash with oil and then add the water. Sprinkle salt and pepper over the casserole, cover, and then bake for 1 hour, turning the meat and vegetables regularly.

Serve on its own or with green vegetables and perhaps some couscous (see page 172) or brown rice (see page 177).

Jamie's osso bucco with parsnip mash   serves 2

This dish is from my nephew, Jamie Sach. It is a great winter dish for people who need iron for energy to play sport and exercise – and who like something tasty and healthy. Parsnips are an underrated root vegetable, and whether roasted or mashed with potato, they benefit the spleen and pancreas (excellent for diabetics) and are high in silicon, which helps to strengthen hair and nails.

2 thick slices beef shin (osso bucco cut)

4 tablespoons plain flour

sea salt and freshly cracked black pepper, to taste

olive oil, for frying

1 large leek, washed and thickly sliced

2 medium carrots, finely chopped

2 sticks celery, finely chopped

2 tablespoons olive oil

1–1.5 litres beef stock

140 g crushed tomatoes

1 small handful parsley, chopped

2 bay leaves

4 medium parsnips

4 medium waxy potatoes

1 knob butter or margarine

Preheat the oven to 180°C.

Score the edge of the beef shin in several places – this prevents it from contracting when it cooks. Season the flour in a bowl and toss the beef in it until well coated. Heat a little oil in a shallow frying pan, then add the beef and cook until lightly browned. Transfer to a plate.

Add the leek, carrot and celery to an oiled frying pan. Fry until the vegetables soften just a little, then transfer them to a heavy casserole dish. Place the browned beef on top and then add just enough stock to cover all the ingredients. Add the tomatoes, parsley and bay leaves and season with plenty of salt and pepper. Cover and bake for 2–3 hours; when the meat falls from the bone it is ready.

To prepare the mash, peel and roughly chop the parsnip and potato into equal-sized pieces. Bring them to the boil in a saucepan of water with a pinch of salt. Once soft, drain the vegetables well and add the butter/margarine. Season with salt and pepper and mash roughly – it's nice if it still has a little texture.

Serve the osso bucco on the bed of parsnip mash with a green vegetable of your choice – in my house peas are always a winner!

Barramundi, lemon and potato   serves 4

This is a dish for the whole family. Serve with Rice salad (see page 138) or Couscous salad (see page 146) or three steamed vegetables such as spinach, carrots and squash.

4 medium kipfler potatoes (or other waxy potatoes), cut into cubes
½ green capsicum, deseeded and chopped into small cubes
½ red capsicum, deseeded and chopped into small cubes
4 fillets barramundi or pearl perch (180–200 g per fillet)
juice of 2 lemons
sea salt, to taste
1 tablespoon chopped fresh parsley

Preheat oven to 180°C.

Parboil the potatoes for 5–10 minutes until tender. Drain.

In a medium ovenproof dish add the potato and capsicums, then top with the fish fillets. Pour over the lemon juice and season with salt. Bake for 15–20 minutes or until the fish is cooked through.

Remove from the oven and sprinkle over the parsley.

Butterfly zucchini pasta   serves 4

*This is a wonderful dish that I often serve as a dinner-party entrée or when I feel like
a lighter meal. If serving as a light meal, add a lentil or chickpea salad on the side.*

400 g farfalle (butterfly-shaped) pasta
2 tablespoons extra-virgin olive oil
1 medium onion, finely chopped
2 cloves garlic, chopped
2 zucchini, finely sliced
sea salt and freshly cracked black pepper, to taste
grated parmesan, to serve
freshly chopped parsley, to serve

Bring a large saucepan of salted water to the boil. Add the pasta and boil for 6 minutes
or until al dente.

While the pasta is cooking, heat the oil in a frying pan and place over medium heat.
Add the onion, garlic and zucchini and sauté for 2 minutes or until the onion and zucchini
begin to brown, then remove from heat.

Drain the pasta and return it to the saucepan. Mix the zucchini sauce through the pasta
and season with salt and pepper. Stir some parmesan and parsley through and serve.

Jamie's Thai beef salad   serves 2

My nephew Jamie Sach's Thai beef salad contains a wonderful mix of vitamins. Beef is high in vitamin B, folic acid and iron. All the vegetables are high in vitamins A and C, and the coriander and mint aid digestion of the meat and help cleanse the liver. Basil is a herb known to 'lift the spirits'.

1 sirloin steak, fat trimmed
2 tablespoons white rice
coriander sprig, to serve

Dressing
2 cloves garlic, finely chopped
1 small piece lemongrass, finely chopped
1 small piece galangal (or ginger), finely chopped
1 tablespoon sesame oil
juice of 1 lemon
approximately 2 tablespoons fish sauce
1 tablespoon white vinegar

Salad
4 spring onions, finely sliced
1 medium red onion, finely sliced
1 medium carrot, finely sliced
1 small red capsicum, deseeded and finely sliced
1 small green/yellow capsicum, deseeded and finely sliced
1 stick celery, finely sliced
1 bunch fresh coriander, washed and patted dry, leaves picked and roughly chopped
1 bunch fresh mint, washed and patted dry, leaves picked and roughly chopped
1 bunch fresh Thai basil, washed and patted dry, leaves picked and roughly chopped

To make the dressing, combine the ingredients (I like to use a lot of fish sauce, but adjust according to taste – it is quite salty) in a small bowl and mix well. Set aside while you prepare the steak and salad.

Cook the steak on a preheated grill to medium–rare. Remove from heat and set aside to rest.

Place the rice in a dry frying pan and cook over a medium–hot heat until the rice begins to turn toasty brown. Transfer the rice to a mortar and grind it coarsely using a pestle.

To make the salad, place all the ingredients in a large salad bowl and combine well.

Slice the steak into thin ribbons and toss with the vegetables and then add the dressing. Lastly, toss through the crunchy toasted rice. Serve with a sprig of coriander on top.

Spaghetti with garlic, oil and chilli   serves 4

This is a very quick and easy dish to make if you are hungry and need something tasty, light and clean to the palate. It is excellent for those with sensitive stomachs, as well as hungry teenagers and students.

400 g spaghetti
2–3 tablespoons extra-virgin olive oil
4 cloves garlic, chopped
1 fresh chilli, finely chopped
½ bunch fresh parsley, chopped
1 handful parmesan, grated
sea salt and freshly cracked black pepper, to taste

Bring a large saucepan of water to the boil. Add the spaghetti and boil for 6 minutes or until al dente.

While the spaghetti is cooking, heat the oil in a frying pan and place over medium heat for 30 seconds or until the oil is hot. Add the garlic and sauté for 1 minute, then add the chilli and sauté until the garlic is just brown.

Drain the spaghetti and return it to the saucepan. Add the oil and garlic mixture and stir to combine. Add the parsley and parmesan, then season with pepper and salt, stir and serve.

Whole baked snapper   serves 2

Snapper is high in most nutrients, especially vitamin A, which helps if you have dry and flaky skin. This is an easy dish to prepare after a long day at the office, especially on a hot summer evening. Serve with a green salad or steamed vegetables or new potatoes.

2 medium snapper, cleaned and scaled
1 medium onion, finely sliced
1 medium tomato, finely sliced
1 clove garlic, chopped
juice and grated rind of 1 lemon
rock salt and freshly cracked black pepper, to taste
butter, for baking
1 fresh red chilli, finely chopped (optional)

Preheat oven to 180°C.

Rinse the fish under running water and dab dry with paper towel.

Place two large sheets of foil on a baking tray and place each fish on a sheet of foil. Arrange slices of onion, tomato and garlic over each fish and then sprinkle the lemon rind over. Pour the lemon juice over the top and season with salt and pepper. Add a dob of butter to the top of each fish and chilli (if using). Fold foil around the fish so each is enclosed in its own parcel, and bake for 20 minutes. To test whether the fish is cooked, use a fork to gently pull a small part of the flesh away. If the flesh is white and tender, the fish is ready. Serve with Jacket potatoes (see page 166).

Tofu and shiitake mushroom stir-fry   serves 2

This is especially good for those with a lowered immune system. Shiitake mushrooms are a natural source of interferon, a protein that stimulates a positive immune response. They are also known for their ability to lower levels of cholesterol and fats in the blood.

Tofu is very digestible, high in B vitamins and minerals, and is inexpensive and low in kilojoules, as well as being a valuable source of calcium. It should be stored covered with water in an airtight container in the refrigerator; change the water daily. It can be baked, steamed or sautéed and added to any vegetable dish for a light protein.

3 dried shiitake mushrooms

1 cup water

1 tablespoon peanut oil

2 tablespoons sesame oil

1 cup fresh or (defrosted) frozen green peas

1 carrot, grated

1 small onion, chopped (optional)

200 g tofu, cut into small cubes

½ teaspoon rock salt

2 teaspoons soy sauce

1 tablespoon sesame oil

freshly cracked black pepper, to taste

Soak the mushrooms in the water for 20–30 minutes, then drain, reserving and straining the soaking water. Discard the mushroom stalks and thinly slice the mushroom cups.

Pour the peanut and sesame oil into a frying pan over a medium–high heat and add the mushrooms. Sauté for 2 minutes, then add the peas, carrot and onion (if using), and half of the soaking water and cook for 5 minutes on high.

Add the tofu cubes to the cooked vegetables, then the rest of the soaking liquid, salt, soy sauce and sesame oil. Cook for a further 5–10 minutes (do not break the tofu cubes) stirring once or twice.

Season with pepper and serve on rice or with a green salad.

Kebabs   serves 4

This is ideal cooked on the barbecue for eating outdoors in summer. Serve with a green salad for extra nutrition and colour.

your favourite vegetables, such as:
  1 green capsicum
  1 squash
  1 large mushroom
  1 tomato
  1 zucchini and
  1 eggplant, all cut into chunks
8 bamboo skewers, soaked
  in cold water for 20 minutes
  (this will prevent them from
  burning on the barbecue)
100 g fetta, cut into large cubes

1 free-range chicken breast fillet,
  cut into large cubes
1 piece flake or pearl perch,
  cut into large cubes
½ cup extra-virgin olive oil
sea salt and freshly cracked
  black pepper, to taste
4 sprigs fresh mint, ½ bunch
  fresh basil or ½ bunch dried
  oregano, chopped
Tahini (see page 164) or Simple tomato
  sauce (see page 175), to serve

Lightly brush the vegetables, cheese, chicken and fish with oil, then season with salt and pepper. Thread them onto the skewers, alternating ingredients, and then sprinkle with the herbs and chilli (if using). Grill the skewers on a hot plate or barbecue, turning, for 15 minutes or until the chicken and fish are cooked and brown. Serve with tahini or Simple tomato sauce.

Roast spatchcock   serves 4

Rosemary or honey can be used instead of garlic to flavour the spatchcock. For a single person, cooking one spatchcock as a mini-roast is great – you can leave it to cook while you go for a run.

4 free-range spatchcock
4 cloves garlic, chopped
4 medium potatoes, peeled and halved
2 carrots, halved and then sliced lengthways
1 onion, quartered
1 small sweet potato or 200 g pumpkin, peeled and roughly chopped
1 parsnip, peeled, halved and then sliced lengthways
2–3 tablespoons olive oil
sea salt and freshly cracked black pepper
2 tablespoons chopped parsley, to garnish

Preheat oven to 180°C.

You may choose to leave the spatchcock whole or you can use poultry scissors to cut along the breastbone to flatten, giving 2 halves per serve (children may only need half this amount).

Arrange the spatchcock, garlic, potato, carrot, onion, sweet potato or pumpkin and parsnip in a large baking dish. Sprinkle the oil over the spatchcock and vegetables and then season with salt and pepper.

Bake for 1–1½ hours, turning the spatchcock and vegetables 2–3 times so that they cook evenly.

When the spatchcock and vegetables are cooked (to test the spatchcock, insert a skewer into the thickest part of the leg – if the juices run clear and there is no blood, the spatchcock is ready), increase the oven temperature to 250°C for 5 minutes, to brown the potatoes.

Remove the baking dish from the oven and drain the spatchcock and vegetables on a paper towel. Serve garnished with parsley.

Vegetable rissoles   makes 12 rissoles

Rissoles are a clever way to encourage the family to eat a range of vegetables. Potato is a great base to start with, but you can also try rice or buckwheat if you are feeling a little more adventurous.

If you have leftover vegetables in your refrigerator at the end of the week, rissoles are a good way of using them up – be creative! Tahini (see page 164) can be added for extra taste, as well as herbs such as basil or thyme.

4 medium potatoes, peeled and cut into quarters

200 g pumpkin, peeled and cut into quarters

240 g frozen peas

1 teaspoon unsalted butter

olive oil

1 medium onion, finely chopped

2 zucchini, finely chopped

2 medium carrots, finely chopped

2 free-range eggs, beaten

1 cup fresh wholemeal breadcrumbs

3 tablespoons chopped fresh parsley

1 teaspoon sea salt

Place the potatoes and pumpkin in a large saucepan and cover with water. Bring to the boil over high heat, then reduce heat to low and simmer for 15 minutes or until the potatoes and pumpkin are cooked. (You may prefer to steam the vegetables.)

Meanwhile, place the peas in a separate saucepan and cover with water. Bring to the boil over high heat and cook for 5–10 minutes or until the peas are soft.

Drain potatoes, pumpkin and peas and combine in a large mixing bowl. Add the butter and mash the vegetables together.

Add a little oil to a large frying pan over medium heat. Add the onion, zucchini and carrot and sauté for 5 minutes. Transfer the mixture to the bowl of mashed vegetables, then add the eggs, parsley and salt and mix well. When the mixture is cool enough to handle, shape it into patties with your hands, then roll them in breadcrumbs to thoroughly coat. Refrigerate the rissoles for 1 hour.

Preheat oven to 180°C.

Place the rissoles on an oven tray lined with baking paper and bake for 30–40 minutes or until brown. (You may prefer to pan-fry the rissoles for 5 minutes on each side.) Serve with your favourite salad.

Fish with soy sauce and ginger serves 2

This is a great recipe for the whole family. I often make this dish after work because it is quick and easy. Ginger helps digestion, but you can substitute some parsley or coriander or finely chopped garlic if you prefer. Tamari is a wheat-free soy sauce, which can be bought in a health store. Look for salt-reduced soy sauces if you suffer from fluid retention or cardiovascular disease.

2 fillets mahi mahi or your favourite boneless fish
1 teaspoon finely chopped fresh ginger root
2 tablespoons tamari
juice of 1 lemon
2 tablespoons olive oil

Cut the fish into 2 cm squares. In a bowl, combine the ginger, tamari and lemon juice. Add the fish and allow it to marinate for 30 minutes.

Heat the oil in a frying pan over medium heat. Add the fish and marinade and cook, stirring gently, for 5–8 minutes or until the flesh is white and soft.

Serve on a bed of Couscous (see page 172) or Mashed potato (see page 176) and a salad of freshly chopped rocket.

CHICKEN DRUMSTICKS

Here are my two favourite recipes for chicken legs, which make a wonderful snack for children when they get home from school or served cold as part of their school lunch, and also for parties when you are feeding a large number of people – just double or triple the quantities. You can also serve these with Jacket potatoes (see page 166), Caesar salad (see page 148) or any other salad.

Honey soy chicken drumsticks   serves 4

½ cup soy sauce

½ cup honey

8 free-range chicken drumsticks

1–2 tablespoons sesame seeds (optional)

1–2 tablespoons pumpkin seeds or cashew nuts (optional)

Preheat oven to 180°C.

In a jug combine the soy sauce and honey. Place the chicken drumsticks in a large baking dish and pour the marinade over them.

Transfer the chicken drumsticks to a baking dish and sprinkle over the sesame seeds, pumpkin seeds and cashew nuts (if using). Bake, turning the chicken drumsticks every 15 minutes, for 1 hour, or until they are crisp and brown.

Chicken drumsticks with rosemary and chilli   serves 4

1½ cups dry white wine

3 cloves garlic, chopped

1 tablespoon fresh rosemary

½ teaspoon chilli flakes or powder

8 free-range chicken drumsticks

¼ bunch parsley, finely chopped

Preheat oven to 180°C.

In a jug combine the wine, garlic, rosemary and chilli. Place the chicken drumsticks in a large baking dish, pour the marinade over and cover the dish with foil.

Bake the chicken drumsticks, turning them every 15 minutes, for 30 minutes and then remove the foil and bake for a further 30 minutes, or until they are crisp and brown. Sprinkle the parsley over the chicken to serve.

Butter bean rissoles   serves 2–4

The butter bean is a complete protein that strengthens the liver and lungs. It is also high in potassium and folic acid, and has no cholesterol. Lima beans can help alleviate heartburn, an irritable bowel and arthritis.

2 free-range eggs, beaten
1 cup fresh breadcrumbs
1 large potato, peeled and boiled
1 medium onion, finely chopped
1 medium carrot, finely chopped
2 sticks celery, finely chopped
1 × 400 g can butter beans, drained and mashed
sea salt and freshly cracked black pepper, to taste
vegetable oil, for cooking
2 tablespoons finely chopped fresh mint or parsley

Place the eggs and breadcrumbs in separate bowls.

In a large bowl combine the potato, onion, carrot, celery, and butter beans. With a masher (or a fork) mash the ingredients and season with salt and pepper.

With wet hands, shape the mixture into patties, then dip each in the egg and roll in the breadcrumbs to thoroughly coat.

Add a little vegetable oil to a frying pan over low heat and cook the rissoles for 2–3 minutes on each side or until brown. Sprinkle with mint or parsley and serve with a rocket or tomato salad.

Lamb and lentils on a bed of mashed potato   serves 4

This is an excellent protein dish for sportspeople, those recovering from illness, or those who need extra body warmth in winter. It is high in minerals, particularly iron.

extra-virgin olive oil, for cooking
1 large onion, roughly chopped
500 g minced lamb
1 medium green capsicum, deseeded and roughly chopped
1 × 400 g can diced tomatoes
1 cup red lentils
3 cups water or Vegetable stock (see page 159)
2 teaspoons chilli paste (optional)
3 teaspoons mixed dried herbs
sea salt and freshly cracked black pepper, to taste
Mashed potato (see page176)

Heat a little oil in large saucepan over low heat. Add the onion and cook until it is translucent and soft. Add the lamb a little at a time, constantly stirring to break up any lumps. When all the lamb is browned, add the capsicum, tomatoes, lentils, water, chilli and herbs. Season with salt and pepper, then simmer for 35 minutes.

Serve on a bed of mashed potato with a mixed green salad on the side.

Prawns with Asian herbs serves 4

This is an excellent summer dish, particularly for those who are watching their weight or changing from heavier meat dishes to lighter foods.

1 kg raw prawns
juice of 2 limes
1 stick lemongrass, chopped
1 tablespoon grated fresh ginger
½ fresh chilli, chopped (optional)
½ teaspoon ground turmeric
½ teaspoon ground cumin
1 handful fresh coriander, chopped
2 cups jasmine or basmati rice
2 tablespoons vegetable oil
1 × 325 g can light coconut milk

Shell the prawns, leaving the tails intact. In a large bowl combine the lime juice, lemongrass, ginger, chilli, turmeric, cumin and coriander. Add the prawns, mix well and leave to marinate for 10–15 minutes.

Bring a large saucepan of water to the boil. Add the rice and boil for 10–15 minutes or until just soft.

While the rice is cooking, heat the oil in a deep frying pan over medium heat. Add the prawns and marinade and cook for 4–5 minutes or until they turn pink. Add the coconut milk and stir to heat through. Taste and add more lime juice if necessary. Drain the rice, arrange in serving bowls, and serve the prawns and sauce over the rice.

Salmon rice rissoles   serves 4

These rissoles are a good balance of protein and carbohydrate. The omega-3 fatty acids assist brain development and healthy skin in children, and in adults they benefit arthritis and high cholesterol. You can use tuna if you prefer.

1 cup fresh breadcrumbs
1 × 400 g can salmon, drained
juice of ½ lemon
1 medium onion, finely chopped
3 cups cooked brown rice (see page 177)
2 free-range eggs, beaten
1 large carrot, grated
vegetable salt, to taste
2 tablespoons extra-virgin olive oil

Place the breadcrumbs in a large bowl.

In a separate bowl combine the salmon, lemon juice, onion, rice, egg and carrot, and season with vegetable salt. Mix well and then, using wet hands, shape the mixture into rissoles, then roll in breadcrumbs.

Heat the oil in a large frying pan over low–medium heat. Add the rissoles and cook for 5 minutes on each side or until light brown on the outside. Place the rissoles on paper towel to drain any excess oil before serving them with a Mixed salad with nuts (see page 142) or a salad of your choice.

Spaghetti vongole   serves 4

Spaghetti vongole is light and tasty, and is delicious for lunch with a salad on a hot summer day. It is also especially gentle on the stomach if you are recovering from a big night out. Clams are a light protein.

400 g fine spaghetti
½ cup extra-virgin olive oil
1 medium onion, chopped
3 cloves garlic, finely chopped
1 kg baby clams, soaked in a bowl
    of cold water for 1 hour before cooking
2 glasses dry white wine
2 tablespoons freshly chopped parsley
sea salt and ½ teaspoon freshly cracked black pepper

Bring a large saucepan of salted water to the boil. Add the spaghetti and boil until al dente.

While the spaghetti is cooking, heat the oil in a large frying pan and place over medium heat. Add the onions and garlic and sauté for 1 minute or until brown. Add the clams and wine, cover and cook for 5–10 minutes or until the clams open, then add the parsley and season with salt and pepper. Discard any clams that do not open.

Drain the spaghetti and place in serving bowls, then pour over the clams and cooking juices.

Pumpkin and sage pasta   serves 4

This dish makes a hearty meal with a salad on the side. Pumpkin is high in antioxidants and sage is a wonderful herb for menopausal women, because it balances the drop in oestrogen, helping to lift the spirits. It contains no protein, but you can add almonds to your side salad (see Chickpea and avocado salad on page 151 and Couscous salad on page 146) if required.

400 g penne
500 g pumpkin, peeled and cut into 2 cm cubes
sea salt and freshly cracked black pepper, to taste
½ cup olive oil
2 teaspoons butter
3 leeks, washed, trimmed and thinly sliced
1 bunch fresh sage, washed and leaves picked
2 tablespoons grated parmesan
4 tablespoons fresh ricotta
fresh peas or fresh young cooked beans (optional)

Preheat oven to 180°C.

Bring a large saucepan of salted water to the boil. Add the pasta and boil for 8 minutes or until the pasta is al dente.

While the pasta is cooking, place the pumpkin cubes on an oven tray and sprinkle with salt, pepper and a little of the oil. Bake the pumpkin, turning regularly, for 20 minutes or until it is soft and browned.

Melt half the butter in a saucepan. Add the leek and fry until soft, then add the remaining butter and the sage leaves, and increase heat until the sage leaves curl and become crisp.

Drain the pasta and then return it to the saucepan. Add remaining oil and the leek–sage mixture. (If the pasta is too dry, add a little stock or water.) Stir in the parmesan and season with salt and pepper. Place the pasta in serving bowls and top with the baked pumpkin, dollops of fresh ricotta and fresh peas or beans (if using).

Soy chicken and potatoes   serves 4

This meal is simple, nutritious and tasty.

2 cloves garlic, crushed

⅓ cup soy sauce

4 free-range chicken breast fillets

1 handful pumpkin seeds (optional)

2 teaspoons sesame seeds (optional)

4 medium potatoes, peeled (or just washed) and quartered,
    or 8 new baby potatoes, washed with skins on

2 tablespoons olive oil

sea salt and freshly cracked black pepper, to taste

In a large bowl combine the garlic and soy sauce. Add the chicken and seeds (if using) and mix well to thoroughly coat the chicken, and set aside to marinate for 20 minutes.

Preheat oven to 180°C.

Transfer the chicken to a medium baking dish and pour over the remaining marinade. Add the potatoes and sprinkle them with oil (for flavour and to allow them to brown while cooking).

After 25 minutes, the chicken should be cooked, so remove from the dish and set aside, keeping warm, leaving the potatoes to cook for a further 20 minutes. Season with salt and pepper and serve with steamed peas, beans and carrots.

Pearl perch with Corn Flakes crusty coating   serves 4

A perfect lighter meal in the evening and for summer, this is excellent for weight loss and joint problems. Children love eating fish cooked this way – it is quick, easy and tasty.

2 free-range eggs, beaten

3 cups Corn Flakes

4 pearl perch fillets, pin-boned

1–2 tablespoons olive oil

2 tablespoons finely chopped fresh parsley

Place the beaten eggs in a bowl. Place the Corn Flakes in a separate bowl and crush coarsely.

Use paper towel to dry the perch. Dip each fillet into the egg, then roll in the Corn Flakes, coating thoroughly.

Heat the oil in a frying pan over low–medium heat for 10–20 seconds. Add the perch fillets and fry for 4–5 minutes on both sides or until cooked and golden brown.

Garnish with parsley and serve with your favourite salad or vegetables.

Lamb casserole   serves 4

This warming casserole for autumn and winter is packed with goodness. It is especially good after a severe virus, flu or cold. The cooking juices are full of vital nutrients, vitamin B_{12}, folic acid and iron from the meat.

2 medium carrots, roughly chopped

2 medium onions, roughly chopped

4 medium potatoes, peeled and roughly chopped

2 medium tomatoes, roughly chopped

2 medium zucchini (or a handful of green beans), roughly chopped

2 cloves garlic, finely chopped

1 teaspoon fresh rosemary leaves

8 lamb (leg) chops, excess fat removed

sea salt and freshly cracked black pepper, to taste

2 tablespoons olive oil

½ cup chopped broccoli and ½ cup chopped cauliflower (optional)

Preheat oven to 190°C.

Add all the vegetables, garlic, rosemary and chops to a baking dish. Sprinkle salt and pepper and pour over enough water to cover the meat and vegetables; about 1½ cups. Pour over the oil and then bake for 45 minutes. Remove from the oven and stir in the broccoli and cauliflower. Continue baking for a further 15–20 minutes.

Serve the casserole by itself or over Couscous (see page 172).

Kingfish with fresh mint sauce   serves 4

This is a very healthy and quick fish dish. It is excellent for weight loss, assists digestion, and the mint helps the breakdown of the essential omega-3 fatty acids. You can also try this dish with marlin instead of kingfish.

4 kingfish fillets, pin-boned
1 teaspoon sea salt
2 tablespoons extra-virgin olive oil
2 large onions, chopped
2 bunches fresh mint leaves, chopped
2 tablespoons white-wine vinegar

Lightly spread salt evenly over both sides of the kingfish. Place the fish under a hot grill and cook for 3–5 minutes on each side.

As the kingfish is cooking, heat the oil in a frying pan over medium heat. Add the onion and mint, and sauté for 5 minutes or until the onion has caramelised. Add the white-wine vinegar.

Arrange the kingfish on serving plates, spoon the fresh mint sauce over it, and serve with your favourite salad or vegetables.

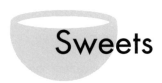

Sweets

Apricot coconut balls makes approximately 12

Like all dried fruit, these are very sweet and should be used only as a small treat. This recipe is not suitable for people suffering from hyperglycaemia or for those trying to lose weight. Apricots are high in copper and cobalt, which assist anaemia.

1 cup dried apricots (or dates or prunes)
1 teaspoon finely grated orange rind
½ teaspoon lemon juice
1 tablespoon orange juice
1 cup desiccated coconut

Soak the apricots in boiling water until they are soft, then drain and finely chop them and transfer them to a large bowl. Add the orange rind, lemon juice and orange juice and mix well. With your hands, form the mixture into small balls and then roll in coconut to coat. Serve immediately or store in an airtight container in the fridge for up to 7 days.

Poached pears   serves 4

The cooking process removes acid and makes fruit very digestible. It is particularly good for the young and elderly with delicate digestive systems or joint problems, and for those with constipation and bloating. I highly recommend homemade cooked fruit for women when they crave sugary snacks.

You can poach or stew any fruit, especially apples and stone fruit such as peaches, apricots and nectarines. You do not need to add sugar. (For fruits other than pears, the vanilla bean and cinnamon stick are optional.)

4 pears, peeled and quartered lengthways (or left whole if you prefer)
1 vanilla bean
1 cinnamon stick
yoghurt or ice-cream, to serve (optional)

Place the pears in a saucepan and cover them with water. Place the vanilla bean and cinnamon stick in the water and simmer for 15–20 minutes, or until soft. Discard the vanilla bean and cinnamon stick, and serve the poached pears plain or with yoghurt, soy ice-cream or a sprinkle of cinnamon.

Anzac biscuits   makes 20 biscuits

What would a nutritious recipe collection be without the famous Anzac biscuits we were all brought up on? They are delicious and filled with rolled oats, which help feed and strengthen the nervous system, and the natural sweetness of golden syrup. These are a far better snack than chocolate, lollies and biscuits. Children love to take them to school as a snack.

1 cup organic rolled oats
¾ cup desiccated coconut
1 cup plain flour (you can use wholemeal, white or gluten-free flour)
1 cup brown sugar
125 g butter
1 tablespoon golden syrup
2 tablespoons boiling water
1½ teaspoons bicarbonate of soda

Preheat oven to 160°C and line 2 oven trays with baking paper.

In a bowl combine the oats, coconut, flour and sugar and make a well in the centre.

In a saucepan combine the butter and golden syrup and place over low heat to melt. In a separate small bowl pour the boiling water onto the bicarbonate of soda to dissolve, then pour this mixture into the melted butter and golden syrup.

Pour the liquid mixture over the oats mixture and stir until combined. Place dobs of the mixture evenly on the oven trays and then flatten a little with your fingers. Bake for 20 minutes and then allow the biscuits to cool on the oven tray for a few minutes before transferring them to a wire rack to cool completely. You can keep leftovers stored in an airtight container for up to 2 weeks.

Baked apples and pears   serves 4

Baking or boiling fruit is one of the best ways to give your family healthy, satisfying, sweet desserts that are not only easy on the digestion but will suit all ages. Cooked fruits are especially wonderful in winter. They are useful for those who suffer heartburn, ulcers, constipation and also help to satisfy the sugar cravings of women with PMT.

1 heaped tablespoon raisins
1 handful almonds, finely chopped
4 apples or pears, cored
1 tablespoon ground cinnamon
2 cups water
yoghurt or soy ice-cream, to serve

Preheat oven to 180°C.

In a bowl combine the raisins and almonds. Stuff the apples or pears with the mixture and sprinkle with cinnamon. Place the fruit in a small baking dish and pour over the water. Bake for 20 minutes or until soft, then serve the fruit with yoghurt or soy ice-cream.

Baked sweet bananas with cinnamon   serves 4

This is one of my favourite desserts, especially on a cold winter evening. Bananas are gentle on the digestive system. They help to detox the body and assist those with a sweet tooth to stop eating sweet junk food. Bananas are especially good for women with PMT who crave sugars, and they are rich in potassium, which is useful for those who play a lot of sport. Cinnamon also warms the blood and assists in digestion. Children usually love this dish.

4 bananas
2 tablespoons brown sugar
½ teaspoon ground cinnamon
¼ teaspoon ground nutmeg
juice and grated rind of 1 orange
1 tablespoon honey or golden syrup
juice and finely grated rind of 1 lemon
2 tablespoons desiccated coconut
yoghurt or ice-cream, to serve

Preheat oven to 180°C.

Peel the bananas, slice them lengthways and place them in a baking dish.

In a small saucepan combine the sugar, cinnamon, nutmeg, orange juice and rind, honey or golden syrup, and the lemon juice and rind. Heat for a few minutes, then pour the syrup over the bananas.

Bake the bananas for approximately 15 minutes or until golden brown and soft, spooning over the syrup every 5 minutes. Remove from the oven and divide among serving plates. Sprinkle the coconut over the bananas and serve with yoghurt or ice-cream.

Index

General

Recipes